Praise for *Enlightened Aging*

"This uplifting account of what it takes to be prepared for an enlightened old age is a must-read for all of us. It translates scientific research on aging to useful advice on building the physical, mental, and emotional reserves to help us age as we most desire."
—**Karen Davis**, PhD, Eugene and Mildred Lipitz Professor; director, Rogert C. Lipitz Center For Integrated Health Care at Johns Hopkins Bloomberg School of Public Health

"We all share the same two goals for our personal end game—a long life and one that preserves our vitality until the end. Yet information on how to achieve those goals is cluttered, confusing, and replete with overhyped promises. *Enlightened Aging: Building Resilience for a Long, Active Life* cuts through the clutter and offers sound, evidence-based advice from a wise physician and geriatrician. Dr. Eric B. Larson offers no magic bullets, but he does present a wealth of common sense that will help you and your loved ones face the inevitable medical, social, and economic choices that come with aging. Spoiler alert: continued physical activity is the next best thing to that elusive magic bullet."
—**Steven A. Schroeder**, MD, distinguished professor of health and health care, University of California, San Francisco; former president and CEO, the Robert Wood Johnson Foundation

ENLIGHTENED AGING

ENLIGHTENED AGING

Building Resilience for a Long, Active Life

Eric B. Larson, MD, and Joan DeClaire

ROWMAN & LITTLEFIELD
Lanham • Boulder • New York • London

Published by Rowman & Littlefield
An imprint of The Rowman & Littlefield Publishing Group, Inc.
4501 Forbes Boulevard, Suite 200, Lanham, Maryland 20706
www.rowman.com

86-90 Paul Street, London EC2A 4NE

British Library Cataloguing in Publication Information Available

Library of Congress Cataloging-in-Publication Data

Names: Larson, Eric B., author. | DeClaire, Joan, author.
Title: Enlightened aging : building resilience for a long, active life / Eric B. Larson,
   MD and Joan DeClaire.
Description: Lanham : Rowman & Littlefield, [2017] | Includes bibliographical
   references and index.
Identifiers: LCCN 2017001674 (print) | LCCN 2017018963 (ebook) | ISBN
   9781442274365 (cloth : alk. paper) | ISBN 9781538174197 (paper : alk. paper) |
   ISBN 9781442274372 (electronic)
Subjects: LCSH: Aging. | Aging—Physiological aspects. | Older people—Health and
   hygiene.
Classification: LCC QP86 (ebook) | LCC QP86 .L365 2017 (print) | DDC 612.6/7—
   dc23
LC record available at https://lccn.loc.gov/2017001674

♾️™ The paper used in this publication meets the minimum requirements of
American National Standard for Information Sciences—Permanence of Paper
for Printed Library Materials, ANSI/NISO Z39.48-1992.

CONTENTS

FOREWORD

H. Gilbert Welch, MD

When I first met Eric Larson, he was a lot older than me. He was a professor of medicine at the University of Washington. I had just finished my residency at the University of Utah and had been hired on as his research assistant. That's a big gap.

Nearly thirty years have passed since then. Now Eric is a hell of a lot older than me. He's in his seventies; I'm still thirty. As you might imagine, confabulation is one of my cognitive issues; I can't remember the others.

Maybe that's why Eric wanted me to read *Enlightened Aging*—particularly the chapter on acceptance.

Aging has been a constant of human experience over the millennia. What's changed is the number of people recommending things that you should do about it. Or, more precisely, things you should purchase for it. The messaging is everywhere: take a medicine, buy some supplements, apply a cream or magnetic field, make appointments to see any number of traditional or alternative health care providers, get tested for x, y, and z. In fact, get tested for anything you *can* be tested for.

But, as you will see, the path to healthy aging is not centered on the consumption of health care services. The path is instead centered on developing the ability to adapt to changing circumstances—the ability to bounce back from an illness, injury, loss, or any other setback. In a word, *resilience*. Don't be fooled by the ads. You don't procure resilience; you build it.

That's what this book is about.

It begins with what Eric calls proactivity. You might think this is a call to avoid inactivity, but that comes later. Instead, it's a call to avoid passivity—particularly when it comes to health care decision making. Get engaged. Get informed. Recognize the strong forces promoting more health care. And recognize that more health care is not necessarily better for you. Develop a little healthy skepticism about health information and make decisions that are right for you. You need to take charge.

The book ends with how to fill three reservoirs: your mental, physical, and social reserves. Think of this as filling a savings account—or filling the woodshed for the impending winter. You want to have a little excess capacity; having reserves is critical to adapting to the changing circumstances that accompany aging. So keep learning new things, keep moving, and keep connecting with others. It doesn't have to be complicated. An engaging conversation during a brisk walk (preferably on uneven surfaces) with a close friend can do the trick.

In between, Eric explores the importance of acceptance. This is the chapter I most needed to read. (Eric, born in 1946, is on the leading edge of the baby-boom generation. I'm near the end of it.) You don't need to dwell on aging, but don't deny it either. That's a recipe for disappointment, discouragement, and unhappiness. Eric accepts he's not going to climb Mount Rainer again, but he has discovered other ways to meet his love for challenging outdoor activities. I've never climbed Rainer (or anything close to the nine thousand feet of vertical gain). But I love the outdoors too and see the value of moderating my view of what constitutes challenging physical activity.

Acceptance of aging calls for more broad-based moderation: how many tasks we expect to do in a day, how many people we need to see, how much to cram into our schedules. In short, moderating our expectations. Ironically, this may be central to our happiness (and, in turn, our health). How we feel about experiences has something to do with what we expected in the first place. While there is certainly a case for having high expectations (particularly for the young), I believe there is also a case for lowering expectations. The reason is simple: high expectations are hard to meet, and lowering expectations makes successes more possible. Of course, there's a balance: challenge yourself, but make sure the challenge is adjusted for age. Avoid the attendant downsides of high expectations—disappointment, discouragement, and un-happiness.

One more thing to accept: There are no guarantees in life (except death). You can be proactive, have your reserves overflowing, and still experience an event you can't bounce back from. In other words, good people doing all the right things nevertheless may experience bad events. This book is not about guarantees; it's about how to stack the odds in your favor.

Eric is well placed to write about these issues. He started thinking about aging when he was young. In 1986, he took the idea of a cancer registry and applied it to patients with Alzheimer's disease—well before the disease was the focus of public (and even medical) attention. The Alzheimer's Disease Patient Registry established how variable the disease was in different patients and began to explain why some patients progress more slowly than others. He then took the idea of the Framingham Heart Study (a population-based cohort exploring the risk factors for heart disease) and applied it to community-dwelling older adults to learn about the risk factors for developing Alzheimer's Disease. In the ensuing pages, you learn a lot more about the Adult Changes in Thought (ACT) study.

And Eric's expertise goes well beyond cognition. He is a practicing general internist—that's a primary care doctor for adults. He understands the other challenges that can accompany aging, things like heart disease, cancer, arthritis, and depression. He's also an administrator, a teacher, and a research mentor. He taught me how to do research, how to write, and how to be understood by others. I am indebted to him.

That's why I wrote this foreword.

That and the fact I knew I was aging and needed to read the book. Maybe you should too.

—H. Gilbert Welch, MD, professor of medicine,
Dartmouth Institute for Health Policy and Clinical Practice

INTRODUCTION

Why "Enlightened" Aging? And Why Now?

As a physician-scientist, I have wanted to publish a book for mainstream audiences about our discoveries in healthy aging for a long time. And now that this project has come to fruition, I realize our timing could not have been better. What a unique era this is! Peak numbers of baby boomers are starting their retirement years just in time to benefit from the emerging science of healthy aging. Never before have so many people lived to be ninety, ninety-five, or one hundred years old. And never before have so many people in late middle age had the chance to learn so much about growing old from their elderly parents' experience. If ever there was a time to become enlightened about our prospects for a healthy old age, it is now.

These lessons come with great urgency—especially considering the huge demographic wave that is already sweeping our nation. This force will only become more powerful with time. The U.S. Census Bureau predicts that the population aged sixty-five to eighty-nine will double between 2010 and 2050. Meanwhile, the number of people ninety and over will more than quadruple.[1]

The implications of this shift are unknown because nothing like this has ever occurred before. Most forecasters are beset with worry and expect unprecedented difficulties for societies and individuals. But I hold a different view. Mine is optimistic, based on many factors. One is my experience studying and caring for thousands of elderly people who embrace aging with resilience and equanimity. The other is faith in my own generation and its proclivity for activism, problem solving, and community building in the face of any number of challenges. Add to this our growing scientific understanding of how to prevent or postpone age-related illness and disability, and I see that boomers have many reasons to expect a better experience of aging than their parents' generation had.

Of course, I haven't always had this optimistic view of aging. In fact, when I took my first foray into geriatrics research in 1978, this whole business seemed rather mysterious (albeit fascinating) to me. I had been hired as medical director of the new University of Washington (UW) Geriatric and Family Services Clinic, founded by psychiatrist Burton Reifler. It was a dynamic time for the field as we were just beginning to realize the significant effects that various forms of dementia—and Alzheimer's disease in particular—would soon have on our aging society. There were lots of "firsts." For example, the husbands of two of our original patients established the first self-help group for caregivers of people with dementia, a movement that eventually led to the formation of the national Alzheimer's Association.

We were also discovering just how much we had to learn. I had recently completed a chief residency in internal medicine at UW Medical Center and felt rather confident in my knowledge and abilities. But in our newly formed clinic, I was quickly humbled by what I didn't know. This awareness drove me to the library, where I read everything I could find about the scientific underpinnings of gerontology and geriatrics. But in working with patients and families, I realized most of what I had learned in medical school, in my training, and from the journals didn't correspond to what we were finding in clinical experience. So we began to collect observational data and publish scientific papers about our findings. This led to research grants, launching our careers in research on aging.

Fortunately, I had been part of the Robert Wood Johnson Foundation's Clinical Scholars Program, which included training in the science of epidemiology at UW's School of Public Health and Community Medicine. Our focus included chronic disease epidemiology—that is, the study of long-term conditions that predominantly affect older people. One key lesson was the importance of studying chronic diseases as they occur in general populations rather than studying them only among people who have been referred to specialty clinics for care of specific conditions. This helped me understand the gaps in my education to date. My training had been based on research in specialized, referral populations—mostly in younger people with rare conditions, not the kind of people we were seeing in our newly formed clinic. Previous findings didn't reflect most people's experience with Alzheimer's disease and other dementias. Going forward, we could look for opportunities to fill this breach.

With this background, my colleagues and I received an award from the National Institute on Aging (NIA) to develop an Alzheimer's disease patient registry—the kind of resource cancer researchers have long used for systematically collecting data among larger, more generalizable populations. Our partner would be Group Health Cooperative, a large Seattle-based health plan that provided comprehensive health care and coverage for hundreds of thousands of people in Western Washington. With access to Group Health members' medical records and other data, we would be able to capture nearly 100 percent of each study participant's care experience. This would give us a better window into how large, broad-based populations were experiencing dementia and other age-related conditions.

NIA awarded our first grant for the UW/Group Health Alzheimer's Disease Patient Registry (ADPR) in 1986 and has continued to support our research ever since, including our future work through 2020. With these funds we developed the Adult Changes in Thought (ACT) study, one of the longest-running community-based studies of Alzheimer's disease dementia, memory, and thinking. The longitudinal nature of the study, funded for more than twenty years, has resulted in a unique resource for studying large numbers of people aging to eighty-five, ninety, and beyond.

Because our work is embedded in a real-world population, many of our discoveries have been quite practical—the kind of knowledge people can use in their everyday lives to prevent illness, care for age-related conditions, and build resilience for a long, active life. That's what motivated me to write this book. I want to share our discoveries—along with other important scientific findings—to help people everywhere improve their health and prepare for the changes that aging brings. But of course, knowledge alone is not enough for "enlightened" aging. We must also have the foresight and wisdom to act on what we know. I hope this book will provide you with the inspiration to do just that.

In the pages ahead, you'll have a chance to read about many of these amazing people—as well as several of my own friends, relatives, and colleagues who have generously shared their stories with us. To protect their privacy, we have changed many of their names and a few identifying details. Still, I trust that their generous participation in this project will inspire you as much as their strength and spirit have inspired me.

—**Eric B. Larson**, MD

I

WELCOME TO THE AGE OF ENLIGHTENMENT

The year was 2006, and phones at our research center were ringing nonstop. Journalists from around the world were calling to confirm the news: we had identified a key factor in staving off some of the most feared conditions of aging—Alzheimer's disease and related dementias.

The discovery had been a long time coming. Human beings have been looking for an answer to age-related brain dysfunction since before Ponce de Leon scoured the New World looking for the elusive Fountain of Youth.

But our findings had nothing to do with healing waters. We weren't even offering a pill. Our solution: regular exercise for at least fifteen minutes, three times a week.[1]

"That's it? Fifteen minutes? Three times a week?" The TV news producer sounded skeptical.

"More activity is better," I told her. "But our study of seniors showed that even small amounts make a difference. And we found that the more frail a person is, the more he or she may benefit from exercise."

"So can we interview one of your study participants on Monday?" she asked.

"No problem," I said. "I'll introduce you to Evangeline Shuler."

"Van," as her friends and family called her, was a delightful one-hundred-year-old who visited our research clinic every two years for checkups. She cheerfully submitted to our study assessments, nailing each challenge we gave her—from memory quizzes to balancing acts to tests of muscle strength and reaction time. Always smiling and sociable with the study team, she was the perfect ambassador for our research. I asked one of our staff to give her a call.

But there was a problem. "That sounds like something I'd like to do," said Van, who always seemed up for an adventure. "But I'll be in Buenos Aires on Monday. I'm going to the annual tango festival!"

Intrigued, the news crew changed their schedule to meet Van at our clinic that afternoon. She arrived via her usual mode: traveling alone by city bus. Once there, she was happy to answer all the reporters' questions. Then she donned her dancing shoes and demonstrated her favorite moves for the television cameras.

Remarkably, Evangeline Shuler lived *another seven years* after that interview. But perhaps even more impressive than her longevity was the way she had lived. From her young adulthood as a social worker among poor immigrants in Chicago's famous Hull House to her postretirement volunteer service with the Salvation Army in Seattle decades later, she dedicated her life to others.

Late into her years, Van remained doggedly independent, living in a downtown high-rise near Seattle's famous Space Needle. From there, she could walk to weekly dances the city sponsored for seniors at Seattle Center. But because that was not enough socializing for her, she also rode the bus to other senior dances in the suburbs.

A former Peace Corps volunteer, Van loved to travel. She logged 114 tours with the adventure company Road Scholar, formerly known as Elderhostel. River cruises in foreign lands were her favorite. Her daughter Lynn Chalmers recalls watching her pack mosquito netting for her trip down the Amazon River. "She wanted to be out on the deck—not inside. She had this wonderful curiosity. She would enmesh herself in the scenery or whatever the guides were talking about."[2]

Lynn observed her mother's optimism and resilience through good times and bad. "She lost many people as she grew so old. But this was her secret: make new friends!" Van had a knack for initiating conversations, getting people to talk about themselves, Lynn explained. "People thought the world of her because they were able to tell her their own stories."

Van's willful adaptability served her well even as her vision diminished with age. Once an avid reader, she switched to books on tape when she could no longer read. Her favorite literature? Biographies, of course. Van never tired of listening to the life stories of others.

Eventually, her blindness made living alone impossible. So when she was 102, Lynn and her partner, Bill, invited Van to live with them. Like nearly every elderly person I've met, Van did not want "to be a burden" to her family. And to hear Lynn tell it, she was not.

"We wanted her to be with us," said Lynn. She traveled with the couple to Bill's veterans group reunions. "She was a hit," Lynn remembers. She would strike up conversations with those around her. "Everybody remarked on her age, and they wanted to dance with her."

Maybe that's because they saw Van as a role model. She was active and joyful, surrounded by friends and family, savoring life until the very end.

LAST LESSONS FROM THE GREATEST GENERATION

Examining Evangeline Shuler's life raises the question, how do some people achieve this level of contentment and vitality as they live into very old age?

Although Van was extraordinary, she's among many very old people I've known who kept moving, learning, and connecting with others despite their advanced age. I have met dozens of patients and research subjects in their tenth and eleventh decades who continued to travel, play music, ski, attend church, raise horses, learn new computer programs, host parties, or take on other life-affirming activities right up until weeks before they died. At first glance, you might think they lived "charmed lives"; everything went their way. But dig deeper and you hear about the losses and setbacks common to most people. Van's husband, for example, died at age sixty. Others lost children, some tragically. Many survived war, accidents, job losses, and other misfortunes. And yet they continued to thrive years beyond expectation, drawing universal admiration—and for me, they're a source of wonder.

What makes such long, active lives possible? Is it genetics? Good luck? Healthy habits? A great attitude? A combination of all these things? This question is important on a personal level. As individuals, we want to make all our days as happy and fruitful as possible. And we'd like to help our aging family members and friends do the same.

Learning the keys to successful aging is also important to our communities. Take a look at how our society will age over the next few decades and you may be startled: In developed countries worldwide, people age eighty-five and older (the so-called old-old) are the fastest-growing part of the population. In 1980, there were 720,000 Americans over age ninety. But thanks largely to advances in public health, disease prevention, education, and economic well-being, by 2010 that number had almost tripled to 1.9 million.[3]

While this number is impressive, it will be dwarfed by the demographic tsunami that's about to roll ashore. Born between 1946 and 1964, the baby-boom generation will undoubtedly do what it has always done—create unprecedented social change by virtue of its sheer volume and age-related interests. Consider these U.S. Census Bureau projections: From 2010 to 2050, the U.S. population aged sixty-five to eighty-nine is expected to *double*. In that same period, the total population aged ninety and over will more than *quadruple*. By the 2030s, the United States will see its biggest spike ever in the number of people over age ninety. During that decade, the ninety-and-older population will jump *71 percent*.[4]

On one hand, it's great to know that so many of my generation have so many years to live. On the other, many community leaders are worried. How will we meet the needs of so many elderly? Consider what we know about today's generation of old-old people—that is, the baby boomers' parents. A 2011 study from the National Institute on Aging and the U.S. Census Bureau showed that two-thirds of Americans aged ninety and older had trouble walking and climbing stairs. The same number had trouble doing errands such as going to the grocery store or doctors' appointments. Nearly half had trouble dressing or bathing. And four out of ten had significant cognitive difficulties.[5]

Most boomers don't need to read such studies to understand the challenges that could lie ahead. We've experienced these problems firsthand while caring for our parents and other older relatives and friends. We've seen how even the hardiest people slow down eventually. We've waited patiently for Mom or Dad to climb out of the car, put on a coat, or tie their shoes. We've initiated those tough conversations about relinquishing car keys, taking over financial matters, or selling the family home. Many of us know how difficult it can be to find helpers that our parents can afford and trust. And for those whose relatives have suffered from Alzheimer's disease or other forms of dementia, we understand the sorrow of "the long good-bye"—the slow grief that begins years before a loved one's death, and continues as meaningful connection becomes increasingly difficult.

As difficult as these circumstances have been, they come with a silver lining. By living so long, my parents' cohort (the folks that journalist Tom Brokaw dubbed the Greatest Generation, after all) once again has provided us with a profound gift: the opportunity to learn from its experience. Their struggle this time is not to survive the Great Depression, win a war against Nazi oppression, or prevail in the fight for civil rights. Now the lessons come from the Greatest Generation's unprecedented experience with longevity: they are the first generation ever to experience old age in such great numbers. And as their children, we boomers are learning volumes from our parents' survival into old-old age, followed by their experience of dying.

As a research scientist and a primary-care physician specializing in internal medicine, I have spent much of the last forty years studying the processes of aging. Now, as a son—and an aging boomer—I can see how my generation is using our own experience and our parents' hard-won knowledge to change the way we ourselves will grow very old.

One key lesson I have learned: there is no "magic bullet"—no drug, no supplement, no psychological trick or lifestyle strategy to keep us forever young. Over time, human desire for an antiaging remedy has attracted everyone from unscrupulous snake-oil salesmen to serious researchers studying geroscience (the science of aging and disease) at major universities. One serious example: a University of Washington–based research team conducting studies—with dogs—of a drug that suppresses cell growth, which might or might not be linked to the body's overall aging processes. While intriguing, such science is in its infancy and not at all likely to benefit today's aging boomers. The initial observations that formed the basis for this very credible effort came from research involving worms—which are a lot easier to work with than mammals. But testing the drug in dogs is a huge leap, so the watchwords for this experiment and others like it can only be "stay tuned."

In the meantime, uncertainty about aging—and how its ravages could play out in our own lives—can be frightfully unsettling, making magic-bullet solutions that much more attractive. But what if we had a better understanding of aging? Would that change our perceptions? Could richer knowledge inspire us to take bolder steps toward a healthier, happier old age?

Today's science supports the unsettling truth we've witnessed among our aging friends and relatives: live long enough and you will develop at least some of aging's common pitfalls—challenges such as poor vision, hearing loss, osteoarthritis, cardiovascular problems, greater cancer risk, slower thinking, and so on.

But this doesn't necessarily mean that growing older is one long, inevitable downward slide. On the contrary, our generation has a greater chance of avoiding disability and enjoying more years of health in old age than any previous generation—which presents a truly unprecedented opportunity.

Take Alzheimer's disease and its related dementias, for example. Because more people than ever are living into old age, the sheer number of people with these conditions is growing. At the same time, however, the percentage of people among the very old who suffer from these conditions is dropping. Also, an increasingly larger percentage of very old people diagnosed with Alzheimer's disease and dementia are staving off the symptoms until just a year or two before they die.

What's happening here? What's behind this so-called compression of cognitive morbidity into late life? With growing consensus, experts believe this unprecedented (and unexpected) phenomenon is the result of our industrialized society's advances in education, economic well-being, and health care, improved treatment of cardiovascular disease, and reduction in smoking. Many worry that the current obesity epidemic and increasing incidence of diabetes could wipe out these gains for the boomer generation. But we can derive great hope from the fact that healthier lifestyles, improved health care, and better overall living conditions over a life span can turn the tide on an age-related illness as devastating as Alzheimer's disease. It shows that individuals can take steps to prevent or postpone disability until later in late life.

And given that we now have the advantage of learning from the experiences of our parents' generation, I am confident that we can benefit immeasurably from the insights we're acquiring. Add to this discoveries being made in the relatively new scientific fields of geriatrics and gerontology. The result? An approach that combines knowledge about growing old with the foresight to use that understanding to its best advantage. It's an approach I call *enlightened aging*.

EXPERIENCE BUSTS MYTHS ABOUT AGING

By the time my friend and patient Marcus Aquino arrived at our mid-morning appointment, he had already had a pretty busy day. The retired college administrator and Vietnam veteran had risen early, snapped on his Fitbit, and logged a few thousand steps on his daily walk with his wife, Sandy. Returning home, he prepared a fruit smoothie for his mother and brought it to her along with her medications. He practiced his guitar and made some calls—arranging a golf game and nabbing tickets for a local jazz performance. Then he headed out to my office in downtown Seattle.

At age eighty-two, Marcus is older than my boomer colleagues and patients. But his insights about what it takes to stay healthy and happy make him a poster child for enlightened aging. For one, he knows just how long life can be. His dad, a postal worker and vegetable farmer who often worked seven days a week, lived to ninety-nine. His mother, a retired editor, is still on email and walking about at 106.

"I want to remain as fit as I can be," he explains. "I want to play golf and do what I want to do for as long as I can."[6] So in addition to daily walks, he goes to a gym three times a week, where he works on strength training and balance. He recently bought new bicycles for himself and Sandy. He loads them on his motorboat for trips to Puget Sound's San Juan Islands.

Marcus is also motivated by his desire to travel. He wants to take his wife to Paris. He lived there decades ago as a single jazz musician. Now that Sandy has retired, he wants to show her the sights. "But I don't want to be in a wheelchair. And I don't want to totter around. I'd like to be able to walk the streets. In order to do that, I have to exercise, I have to keep fit."

He has three children from a previous marriage—all grown, all successful. When he thinks about the years ahead, he says he doesn't want to become dependent on them the way his mother relies on him. "And I don't want to be dependent on my wife either."

Marcus had some health scares in recent years: a mild heart problem, two aneurysms, and bladder cancer. One year posttreatment, the cancer has not returned. He continues his routine of walking, going to the gym, caring for his aged mother.

He's noticing changes that come with age. And while he doesn't want to accept limitations, he thinks it's best to be adaptable. His golf game is one example. "I have to play it differently now. I have to say, okay, I'm not going to hit the ball 280 yards anymore. So I hit it 200 and I change the clubs I use. I focus on what's possible. Adaptability—that's the difference."

Reminded of his age, Marcus seems bemused. "Honestly, this is not how I imagined eighty years old would be," he says. "When I was young, I thought everybody this age would be decrepit, walking around with a cane. But that just hasn't happened to me—yet."

Marcus's experience busts a common myth about aging: there's nothing you can do to avoid disability as you grow old. By staying active and engaged in his life—despite illness and limitation—he's continuing to build strength and well-being. His persistence and adaptability increase the chances he'll soon make that trip to Paris with Sandy—and have many other adventures ahead as well.

Marcus's life also contradicts the myth that people become increasingly miserable as they age. Research shows that many people, both young and old, live with this mistaken belief, causing them to dread the prospect of aging. In a telling 2006 study published in the *Journal of Happiness Studies* (yes, there is such a thing), social scientists asked two groups of adults—one younger (average age thirty-one) and one older (average age sixty-eight)—which of the two groups they *believed* to be happier. As expected, both groups thought the younger people would be happiest. But when they asked both groups to rate their own well-being, they found the older group was the happier bunch.[7]

Many other studies have reached the same conclusion. People in general find more happiness in old age than during their middle years—an idea we'll explore more deeply in chapter 3. But if anybody had told me this at the beginning of my career, I never would have believed it.

PETE TOWNSHEND WAS WRONG

Looking back at my days at Harvard Medical School, I can see how the spirit of the late 1960s and early 1970s influenced me. In an era that celebrated youth above most other values, we boomers made our mark by challenging conventional ideas and behavior. We rejected identities that would anchor us to our elders and their interests. Many of my medical school colleagues and I bought into musician Pete Townshend's estimation that growing old looked awfully cold; we resisted specializing in geriatrics, considering it a dismal pursuit.

And yet the 1970s were a fruitful time for medical researchers interested in the aging brain. Previously, many believed nothing could be done about "senility."

But now bench scientists were beginning to seriously explore various causes of dementia—including both the rare form of Alzheimer's disease that strikes younger people and the more common type that's widespread in the elderly, as well as other conditions that cause serious cognitive decline in older populations.

Also, as we looked into the demographic crystal ball, we could see many pressing health and social services issues on the horizon. Finding ways to better care for a growing elderly population seemed especially appealing to those interested in a meaningful and future-oriented career. In addition, the National Institute on Aging (NIA) was increasing resources for those who wanted to do the research. So in 1978, when I finished my chief residency in internal medicine at the University of Washington (UW) and was offered a chance to help start a new venture, the UW Geriatric and Family Services Clinic, I decided to take the plunge. Little did I know how fascinating I would find the lives of old people and the study of aging.

Founded by then Psychiatry Assistant Professor Burton Reifler, the clinic soon became the first geriatrics research facility in the country to systematically evaluate and study old people living outside of institutions who were thought to have Alzheimer's disease or dementia. Over time, our team began using some of the same research methods—such as patient registries—that have proven successful in the study of cancer. In my role as the clinic's medical director, I worked alongside a psychiatrist and a social worker, assessing patients and documenting our observations. This was long before desktop computers showed up in exam rooms, so we simply collected data on forms we carried in our lab coat pockets. Although rudimentary, the system allowed us to collect the information we needed, analyze our findings, and ultimately share our results with other health professionals and scientists worldwide in scientific journals.

Having specialized in the field of internal medicine—which takes a special interest in the complex diseases of adulthood—I thought I knew quite a lot about old people. But once I started seeing patients in the geriatrics center, talking with their family members, and carefully assessing what was happening in their day-to-day lives, I realized that much of what I had learned about aging in medical school was *just plain wrong*.

Take drugs, for example. At that time (as today), physicians were widely prescribing drugs for controlling the behavioral symptoms of Alzheimer's disease and related dementias. But as we observed in our patients, these pills, which have since been taken off the market, were not working very well at all. Even worse, some prescription drugs taken by our patients for other common chronic conditions of aging, such as hypertension, depression, arthritis, insomnia, and incontinence, caused cognitive impairment overall. The results in many cases were detrimental, and sometimes even dangerous.

I vividly remember one patient whose husband, a physician, had prescribed sedatives to help her sleep. We recommended she quit the sleeping pills, and when she did her confusion and forgetfulness disappeared. It surprised me that this simple change could result in such a dramatic improvement, and yet we saw this kind of "cure" time and time again as people stopped being overmedicated with drugs they did not need. After documenting several cases like this, our team published a paper in 1987 titled "Adverse Drug Reactions Associated with Global Cognitive Impairment in Elderly Persons."[8] Among the hundreds of papers I've published, this one makes me especially proud. Not only did we describe our patients' most common reversible cause of dementia— a problem that literally went away when people stopped taking the drugs—but consumer advocacy groups shared our findings widely, increasing awareness of how missed diagnoses and overprescribing harm the elderly. (Medication problems continue to be a common cause of "reversible dementia" today—a condition that can mimic Alzheimer's but disappears or improves when patients stop taking the drugs.)

Meanwhile, our team was learning the importance of supporting patients' family members and other caregivers. Until that time, most research on care for dementia and Alzheimer's disease had focused on the patient and how to alleviate his or her symptoms. But when we started looking into the caregivers' role, we saw that many lacked the tools and resources they needed to provide safe, effective care.

Some caregivers, for example, resorted to tying patients to their chairs or beds to keep them from wandering. Others responded to their patients' confused mental states by constantly trying to correct them. Such measures often caused patients a great deal of agitation or anger—resulting in even more misery and disability, and making their care more difficult than ever. We knew the caregivers needed new strategies. So over many years we have worked closely with colleagues from the UW School of Nursing to develop new approaches. One intervention, for example, focused on taking patients for daily walks. The research team found that with increased physical activity, patients not only improved their physical function and had less depression; they also were less likely to be placed in nursing homes because of behavioral issues. We also saw how teaching caregivers basic skills—such as avoiding arguments with the patients in their care, or encouraging caregivers to join support groups—could improve the caregivers' well-being, which contributed to better experiences for the patients as well. These results and subsequent research led to what has become known as the Seattle Protocols—an approach that helps families and caregivers address patients' needs without resorting to mind-altering drugs that cause confusion, sleepiness, falls, and fractures.[9]

But perhaps most important, we gradually learned that it's a mistake to look at Alzheimer's disease and related dementias in isolation, as though they come from a single cause. Over time, research teams at UW and elsewhere began to understand that such dementias occur in the context of several conditions common in the elderly, problems such as cardiovascular disease, uncontrolled high blood pressure, and ministrokes. Together, they complicate lives and make brain function worse.

On one level, this evolution in understanding was discouraging because it dashed our hopes for a single "magic bullet" to "cure" Alzheimer's disease; the causes are just too complex. But there's actually a tremendous silver lining in recognizing the strong links between dementia and other common conditions of aging. It means we may be able to actually prevent or postpone countless cases of dementia until very late in life—in much the same way that we have been winning the battle against heart disease. Consider this statistic from the American Heart Association: the United States saw a *29 percent decline* in death rates from cardiovascular disease from 2003 to 2013.[10] This decline, which can be attributed to ongoing efforts to better prevent, diagnose, and treat heart conditions, may be impacting the risk for Alzheimer's disease and dementia as well. Efforts to avoid tobacco, exercise more, and take better care of conditions like high blood pressure, high cholesterol, and diabetes may be turning the tide. Better educational and socioeconomic opportunities, which improve health from birth until late life, are also making a big difference; research indicates that the more you build brain function through challenging mental activity in early life, the more "reserve" you'll have to resist dementia later on. (We'll explore this concept further in chapter 5.)

Of course, all this emphasis on "healthy living"—that is, increasing our physical activity, improving our diets, avoiding smoking, getting an education, and so on—takes control out of the hands of the doctors and the drug companies and puts it squarely in the hands of everyday people as they go about their daily lives. That means that in order to fully benefit from scientific discoveries about preventing dementia and other debilitating conditions of aging, people must be willing to "take charge" of their own well-being and their own habits. (Can the generation that was so enamored of John Lennon's "Power to the People" muster the same enthusiasm today on behalf of their own health? Doing so could make all the difference!)

So while my colleagues and I left medical school believing we might someday discover and prescribe some miracle drug to prevent our patients' long, slow, downward spiral into the misery of old age, I have learned in recent years just how wrong we were! The notion of a magic pill will always be attractive. But not only is there no magic pill on the horizon; helping our patients benefit from the emerging scientific knowledge on healthy aging requires them to embrace self-care more fully than we might have ever imagined. And what if our generation fully commits to this enlightened approach? Then aging won't be nearly so dismal after all.

STUDYING AGING IN A REAL-WORLD POPULATION

Once I realized that my medical training was not aligned with what I was observing in my patients, my research participants, and my own elderly friends and relatives, I became more determined than ever to find answers.

One big problem with early research on Alzheimer's disease and other dementias was our population—it was too narrow! Our research subjects were recruited almost exclusively from university-based medical centers among highly specialized patient groups. This differs from research where participants are randomly selected from large, general populations. As a result, the early work included disproportionate numbers of people afflicted with Alzheimer's disease at a relatively young age, which is actually rather rare. So the participants' experience did not reflect that of older Alzheimer's patients in the "real world." For example, early-onset Alzheimer's disease is believed to be driven much more by genetics than by other lifestyle or environmental causes. By studying only younger people, were we missing clues related to factors such as physical activity, drugs, or other chronic illnesses?

To eliminate this bias in our science, my colleagues and I decided to take a new approach. Beginning in the mid-1980s, we started collaborating with researchers from a large Seattle-based health plan, Group Health Cooperative. With access to Group Health's large, mainstream population, we could identify a randomly selected group of patients aged sixty-five and older and study them over decades. The research program we developed is now called ACT, which stands for the Adult Changes in Thought.[11]

Initially, we focused on just the brain and Alzheimer's disease, but over time we have expanded to explore healthy aging in general. By 2016, ACT had become the world's longest-running longitudinal study of its kind. ACT is unique both for its duration and the detailed information the study participants agree to share about their routine care.

To be invited to enroll in ACT's "living laboratory," people must initially be free from cognitive impairment—that is, without serious problems with memory and thinking. We stay in regular contact with participants over the rest of their lives, evaluating them regularly for changes in brain function and other health conditions. By analyzing the data we collect from this population over the decades, we're learning a tremendous amount about factors that differentiate healthy seniors from those with dementia and other age-related disabilities.

At nearly 101 years old, ACT participant Joe Feldman is an outlier on the healthy side. Over six feet tall, he greets me at the door of his tidy apartment in a parklike senior community in Shoreline, Washington.

The former newspaper editor used to drive to our downtown Seattle clinic for his evaluations, but he gave up his car keys on his one hundredth birthday. "We sold our ancient car," he tells me. "It was a—" he stops, searching for the word. "See, there you are—a bad moment."[12]

But there's no rush. Five or so seconds pass and then he adds, "Toyota! It was a Toyota!" His wife, Lena, ninety-three, chimes in, "It was a Toyota Camry!"

Although Joe's difficulty finding the right word tries his patience, when I ask him about his childhood, he easily accesses old memories. He tells me he was the son of a tailor during the Great Depression. He and his brother helped the family get by, selling razor-blade sharpeners on the streets of New York. His memories of World War II are vivid. He describes the B-26 twin-engine bombers that carried him as a radio operator/gunner in sixty-five missions over Europe during World War II. "I want to be precise," he says. "It was the Army Air Force, but it started out as the Army Air Corps."

But like most elderly people, Joe is challenged to remember the near-term stuff—say, the names of his medications or a person he's just met.

Other than these frustrations, he seems to be taking aging in stride. He's especially proud that he and Lena live independently. They moved to this ground-level, somewhat spacious apartment about seven years ago from an assisted-living facility that featured programs focused on the needs of the elderly.

"It was so boring it drove me nuts!" Joe says, so they moved out.

He likes to spend his time poking around on the computer. He and Lena use it to order groceries, make doctors' appointments, and schedule rides on the senior shuttle. Best of all, Lena reads the New York Times online, increasing the font size for her poor vision. She also is passionate about Scrabble, which she plays on the Internet. Joe says he gets excited when the computer messes up. "I like to find out, 'What's wrong with this damn thing?'"

Joe's interest in problem solving may put him among an elite group some researchers call super-agers—people over eighty-five who show few signs of cognitive decline. But that's just a guess.

He himself seems mystified by his longevity. "It's strange as the dickens," he explains. His mother died of cancer in her sixties, his dad died of a heart attack at seventy-five, and both of his brothers are long gone. But Joe has never had a heart attack, a stroke, or cancer.

"Maybe it's clean living," he speculates. He quit smoking, drinking alcohol, and overeating many years ago. And back when his gait was more steady, he used to take long walks around the shopping mall. To this day, he hates to sit still for too long. Even in the middle of a TV show, he gets up and walks around a bit.

But as interesting as this may be, it's just one man's experience. It doesn't provide definitive clues about how to live a longer, healthier life. That riddle requires us to follow thousands of older people over many years. So that's why we subject study participants like Joe to a variety of mental and physical tests every other year.

After twenty-two years in the study, Joe knows the drill, but that doesn't make it any easier. At this visit, I start by giving him a math problem—"Count back by sevens beginning at one hundred"—and Joe performs quite well.

Then we do a very basic evaluation of short-term memory. I give him three simple concepts—dog, yellow, Pacific Ocean—and ask him to repeat them, which he does with ease. But after I switch subjects and then return to the series a few minutes later, the exercise is no longer stress-free.

"Do you remember the three things?" I ask.

"Here we go again!" he chuckles. "Let's see. It was about the ocean. And there was a color. Green, was it? I forget."

I reassure him that his difficulty is completely normal. It's rare to see anybody over ninety who can remember all three.

Then we move on to the physical assessment. Taking his hand, I test his grip strength and his reflexes. We're looking for signs of Parkinson's disease, Alzheimer's, or other neurological disorders. Fortunately, I find none.

He's seated at his dining room table, and when I ask him to stand up without using his arms to push off the seat, he balks. "I don't think I can."

"You want to try?" I ask him, and he consents. On a count of thee, Joe pushes forward and finds himself fully vertical, steadying himself on my arm. "I did it!" he laughs, genuinely surprised. "Hey! Thank you!"

Then we do a series of walking tests—examining his balance in moves most younger people do effortlessly. Joe, I'm happy to say, takes none of this for granted. He understands that old bones break easily, so falls are one of the greatest risks he and Lena face. As an extra measure of caution, he and Lena typically use walkers to move about the apartment. "I'm chicken-hearted and I like to play it safe," he explains. "One bad fall and we know we're out of business."

"You're smart to do that," I say.

Just before leaving, I reiterate that Joe seems to be doing extremely well—probably better than 90 to 95 percent of people his age.

Lena muses that Joe faced many major stresses in his life—like the missions he flew during the war, for instance. Also, many years ago, they lost a child who was mentally disabled. "So he has had a lot of tension in his life, and it didn't affect him adversely. I don't know how you can explain that."

I suggest that their lives may be a demonstration of "resilience"—the ability to grow stronger in the face of adversity and stress.

"Some people have it and some people don't," Lena quietly observes, and then asks, "I wonder why?"

THE WHOLE PICTURE

It's just the kind of question we've been asking for decades. By embedding our research in a stable, community-based population of more than half a million people who get their care in one health system, we've been able to collect data on all aspects of our participants' health. Our study subjects have generously granted us access to their electronic health records, including information about prescription medications, lab tests, medical diagnoses, and procedures.

ACT participants come to the research clinic every two years for assessments. Or, if they're too frail to travel, an ACT staff member goes to their homes. During these visits, we test the participants' thinking and physical health and find out about habits like exercise and diet. One subset of the population was even given Fitbit-like monitors to wear so that we could record how much time they spend sitting, standing, and engaging in moderate and vigorous activity. Data like this, when correlated with all the other health information we collect, is helping to answer important questions about the impact of physical activity on thinking and other vital functions.

In addition, we ask our study participants for permission to conduct autopsies on their brains after death. As of 2017, more than 650 participants had donated their brain tissue, providing a unique opportunity for scientists to link extensive population-based clinical information with the latest advances in neuroscience.

DNA from participants' blood, brain specimens, and other tissues are contributed to a national repository for research on "whole genome sequencing"—a process that analyzes genetic structures to better understand the foundations of Alzheimer's disease and a whole host of other health conditions.

After more than thirty years, my colleagues and I have amassed a tremendous amount of scientific information. By 2016, we had enrolled more than five thousand participants, documenting more than forty thousand person-years of data. Since 2004, we have kept a steady number of people (two thousand) enrolled in the study and participating in ongoing assessments. About one in five of our study participants has developed dementia. And from autopsies, we've determined that about eight out of ten of our deceased participants who had dementia had Alzheimer's disease, often combined with other age-related degenerative conditions.[13]

Over the years, as some participants develop dementia and others don't, we explore the differences. The result is "a living laboratory" of aging—especially the aging brain. Our research team, in collaboration with other scientists at UW and around the world, is asking and answering questions such as the following:

- Why do some people get dementia while others stay mentally sharp?
- Why do some people's brains show advanced signs of Alzheimer's disease after death—and yet these same people showed no signs of declining mental function or dementia when they were alive?
- Can dementia be prevented by controlling high blood pressure, diabetes, depression, or other chronic illnesses?

- Can certain medications help prevent or stave off problems with memory and thinking?
- What makes older people resilient—that is, able to bounce back from major physical challenges or other upsets?
- Are certain drugs linked to higher risks for dementia?
- Are head injuries in early life associated with dementia later on?
- Can regular exercise reduce the risk of dementia? If so, how much physical activity is needed to make a difference?
- What about education?
- Does staying socially active matter?
- What other steps can we take to help people prevent or stave off dementia and other serious disabilities of old age?

The knowledge gained from this research—along with other discoveries that scientists worldwide are making—gives us optimism and hope for the coming decades. Together we are finding ways to help people use the science of healthy aging to have a better quality of life up until its very end.

This knowledge is one key element in the promise of enlightened aging. The other is having the foresight to use this knowledge to its full advantage as you plan for your own later years.

RESILIENCE AND THE THREE INTERRELATED STRENGTHS OF ENLIGHTENED AGING

It's been a great honor to work with the ACT participants over the years. As you'll soon read, people everywhere are benefiting from the discoveries we're making together.

On a more personal level, I am grateful for all the time I've spent visiting with these folks, listening to their stories. Along with my own elderly patients, friends, and relatives, the ACT participants have enriched my life in ways that are difficult to quantify. I've often thought how each person's life is like an epic novel or a great film, providing us with important lessons in how to live. If we listen carefully to our elders, we can learn how to live happily through life's ups and downs, endure its sorrows, adjust to changes and losses—and in the end, let go of its struggles.

And if my work as a scientist and physician has revealed one quality that's consistent among those who age well and happily, I believe it's this: *resilience*—the capacity to adapt and grow stronger in the face of adversity or stress. Much has been written about the value of resilience in helping people stay healthy or bounce back from illness and other challenges life throws our way. In observing my patients and research subjects, I see people follow three interrelated steps on a PATH to resilience, which I'll describe at length in the coming chapters. These steps are the following:

1. **Proactivity:** Taking charge of your own health and happiness by preventing illness and managing chronic conditions that may develop. It also means learning to be a partner with your health care providers, sharing important decisions, and getting care that's just right for you—that is, not too little and not too much. You'll learn more about these approaches in chapters 2 and 6.

2. **Acceptance:** Knowing change will come with age, which allows you to approach the future with equanimity and mindfulness—in large part by understanding your own values. Research has shown that we generally seek more meaning, fulfillment, and purpose in our lives as we grow older. We want stronger relationships with friends and family. Many of us want to keep contributing to the world through work, volunteerism, and hobbies. And most of us want to stay as independent as possible. As many patients have told me, we don't want to "be a burden to others" in old age. Being open and realistic about the changes that aging brings will help you to keep such values in mind as you plan for the times ahead. We'll explore these concepts more deeply in chapters 3, 7, and 8.

3. **Three Reservoirs:** Building reserves of well-being in three ways—mentally, physically, and socially—for the long, fulfilling road ahead. We'll explore the significance of these interconnected resources in chapter 4. In chapter 5 we'll describe ways to build, protect, and enhance brain function. In chapter 6 you'll learn about building and maintaining physical reserves beyond the brain—including the heart, bones, muscles, vision, and hearing. In chapter 7, we'll discuss strategies for planning to have the

financial means and social resources you may want as you grow older.

The last chapter explores how our attitudes of activation and acceptance can change the way we approach not only aging—but also death itself. I subtitled this part "Your Reward for a Life Well Lived" because that's how I hope the very last years can be for all of us. By taking an enlightened approach, perhaps we'll come to a place where we can just relax and grow very old knowing we are safe, comfortable, and well cared for. That's the ideal anyway, and the way I've seen life and death play out for many of my patients, research subjects, family, and friends.

But first, we have a lot of living to do. For inspiration, I like to think of Evangeline Shuler boarding that plane to the Buenos Aires Tango Festival at age one hundred.

"Once we got there, we hired a man to dance with us," her daughter Lynn remembers and laughs. "It was our little joke: 'We hired a gigolo!' And we sat at these little tables in an old hotel where everything was covered with marble. That band played three sets of music, took a break for drinks, and then played another three sets. Mother and I traded off. She would dance with him and then he would come back and dance with me. She enjoyed it *very, very* much!"

I tried to imagine all the elements that came together for Van to relish this one last trip. There were all those senior dances at Seattle Center that kept her out in the world and up on her feet. There was her interest in others, her sense of adventure, and her willingness to try new things. I think of the financial resources that paid the airfare. And I also think of her friends and family who cared enough to help her make the voyage. Then I wonder, how on earth does a person manage to have their later years play out like that? Let's find out.

2

PROACTIVITY

Aging with an Attitude

Remarkably witty and agile at age one hundred, our research participant Evangeline Shuler was often asked, "What's your secret to living so well for so long?"

"I wish I knew," replied the retired social worker turned tango dancer. "If I did, I'd be a billionaire!"[1]

However, the more we learn about super-agers like Van, the less mysterious their longevity seems. Inherited traits and healthy habits play a part. Exercising regularly, eating a good diet, not smoking, and maintaining social connections are all essential.

But is there some *attitude* beneath it all that helps people build resilience, prevent illness, and manage chronic conditions in old age? I believe so. Simply put, it's an approach to life that says, "I take action on my own behalf. I am a problem solver. I don't give up in the face of difficulties like stress, illness, and disability. Instead, I embrace opportunities to make matters better for myself and for those around me."

I also believe that the boomer generation—with its history of interest in self-actualization and activism—uniquely holds this game-changing attitude in good measure. And while it's still too early to be certain, I predict that this stance will serve many of us well as we live into our eighties, nineties, and possibly beyond.

Much of my optimism comes from observing people like Van, whose life story bears out the advantages of this take-charge approach. From her early career serving the poor in the slums of Chicago to her middle years establishing a library and a fire station in rural Florida—Van was consistently proactive.

By the time she reached retirement in her sixties, service and adventure still called to her. So she and her husband, Gard, joined the Peace Corps and were sent to a village in the Indian state of Maharashtra. They helped residents there build gardens, smokeless stoves, and a water-drainage system. Tragically, after fifteen months, Gard contracted meningitis and died. Van could have given up, but after a short trip home, she went back to India and completed her twenty-seven-month Peace Corps commitment, followed by months of travel in the South Pacific.

"She later said that returning to India was the best thing she could have done," Lynn said. The work gave her purpose and connection to other people, "and that's how she was able to cope with her grief."

Later in life, Van used a similar strategy to stay strong and active in the face of advanced aging. Lynn said her mother made plans each day that would motivate her to get up, get dressed, and get out the door. Maybe this was the "billionaire" scheme that kept her vital over the decades. "She had to think ahead to the friend she was going to meet or the bus she needed to catch," Lynn said.

While in her nineties, Van would meet a group of friends at eight each morning for coffee. There was a ritual quality to the gathering; each person was expected to share a story or tell the "daily joke." The meeting also served as a safety check. If one member didn't show up, the group would contact that person to be sure he or she hadn't gotten sick or taken a fall.

Over many visits to Van's senior community, Lynn saw her mother's friends decline physically with age. "Yet their enthusiasms, laughter, storytelling, and helpfulness to each other continued," Lynn said.

This arrangement did not occur by chance. Nor did anybody outside of the group make it happen for them. They formed the social circle themselves, knowing it was good for them as individuals and for each other. They did it with purpose because that's what activists do. They take action to create the life they want, to meet the goals they're after.

For Van, being an activist involved a hearty dose of socializing. That's good because staying healthy in old age typically requires strong social support. But I've observed super-agers "taking charge" in many other ways as well. Their drive for well-being makes them set a high priority on staying physically active, avoiding unhealthy foods, and not drinking too much alcohol. They consciously try to keep stress to a minimum, and when stress inevitably happens, they manage it through prayer, exercise, meditation, or other activities that enhance self-awareness and promote a more relaxed state. They keep a careful eye on chronic conditions common to aging, such as diabetes, high blood pressure, arthritis, a heart condition, or high cholesterol. And they have a high awareness of ways to prevent illnesses like the flu and accidents such as falls.

In addition, proactive agers can be quite feisty in their relationships with the health care system and health care providers. They are assertive, and not passively accepting of the paternalism that too often characterizes health care. They're the type of patients who show up at clinic appointments with a list of well-researched questions about their complaints and concerns. They've gone online to look for unbiased, credible health information from authoritative sources. They've read books and articles and talked to their friends and family about staying healthy. Because they've given it a lot of thought, they're not afraid to tell the doctor about their goals for getting and staying well. And when it comes time to make a decision about a treatment or surgery, they like to do it from a place of knowledge and forethought. They don't feel good about passively following "the doctor's orders." They want to make sure their care is based on their *own* values. They are not afraid to reject modern medicine's habit of overtreating and overprescribing medication for common health problems. All of this applies to care near the end of life as well. These are the kind of folks who do "advance-care planning." Although fully engaged in living, they've talked to their doctors, friends, and family about the kind of care they'll want—and won't want—when close to death.

But let's be honest. For many people, developing a more proactive attitude toward health and health care doesn't happen automatically. Depending on your life experience, asserting yourself in health care situations may take some serious conscious effort. It may feel awkward to forgo the deferential attitude patients traditionally have toward their doctors. Most health care systems don't encourage such activism, as they are largely geared toward efficiency. Whether consciously or not, the system is built to "serve those providing the services."

Also, changing health habits can require major planning and commitment. (Ask anybody who has quit smoking or lost a lot of weight and kept it off.) Such changes require us to step outside our comfort zones. They may even require us to stand up against traditional norms within our families, our social networks, and the health care system.

And that's where it all gets interesting. Fortunately for the many boomers now in their sixties and seventies, taking a contrarian, subversive, antiestablishment stand seems quite familiar. And that's the reason I'm optimistic about the way my generation will approach growing very old.

TALKIN' 'BOUT MY GENERATION

While living in Boston in the early 1970s, I often came across tattered copies of an underground booklet called *Women and Their Bodies*. Published on stapled newsprint by a group called the Boston Women's Health Collective, it seemed for a while that this 193-page missive could be found everywhere—in dorm rooms, apartments, student lounges, and "New Age" coffee shops. For women coming of age at the dawn of the women's movement, this was a sign of just how much attitudes were changing.

Although the booklet sold for just seventy-five cents, it provided a wealth of information that was hard for lay people to find—especially self-care advice about reproductive health and sexuality, and women's experiences within a male-dominated health care system. The book was as popular with my female med school classmates as it was among other young women in my social circle. Soon retitled *Our Bodies, Ourselves*, it became a charter of sorts for the burgeoning women's health care movement. As of 2015, the book has been updated several times, distributed to millions of people worldwide, and translated into more than thirty languages.[2]

But even as a medical student in 1971, I couldn't ignore the publication's main message: young activist women were taking control of their health and health care as never before. The book's cover—with its photo of female protesters under a banner reading "Women Unite!"— showed solidarity against the paternalism of Western medicine. Young women were determined to become more knowledgeable about their bodies and better empowered to make care decisions according to their own values. They would no longer be passive consumers of the medical-industrial complex.

Nearly half a century later, I still think about *Our Bodies, Ourselves*, the movement it promoted, and the many dramatic social changes that happened as a result. True, widespread access to affordable, legal abortion remains an ongoing concern. But we've seen tremendous progress in women's health care since the 1960s, when abortion was illegal everywhere, credible sex education was nonexistent, and pharmaceutical companies were promoting unproven hormone treatments to keep women "forever young." Examples of progress since then include providing easier access to birth control, giving families alternative choices for pregnancy care and childbirth, and reducing use of hormone treatment after menopause.

Reflecting on these changes, I envision boomers marshaling an equal level of engagement related to aging. Can the generation that produced *Our Bodies, Ourselves* advance an activist approach to health and health care for our *aging* bodies? Our numbers alone portend tremendous social change as we enter our seventies. By the year 2050, the population of Americans aged sixty-five and older is projected to be about 83.7 million, almost double its estimate of 43.1 million in 2012.[3] What if today's generation of aging boomers could take action for better aging in the same way it once stopped an unpopular and disastrous war, fostered the environmental movement, promoted women's rights, gay rights, and civil rights? And what if the changes we promoted rocked today's medical establishment not only for our own well-being, but also for the benefit of the many generations to come?

Considering this possibility, and its inherent counterculture values, I think of people like my cousin Linda Babcock, age sixty-six. She's now a retired elementary school teacher in Bozeman, Montana, where she and her husband, Clark, raised their two children and lived what appeared to be a conventional life. But I also remember how steeped she was in alternative ideas during her college days in Bozeman. Yes, she too read *Our Bodies, Ourselves*.

"I still have it on my shelf," she recently told me.[4] "It was a common voice, giving us information that we couldn't get from doctors or anyplace else." More than forty years later, she figures that voice still influences her family's health and health care.

"My ideas have been so different from my parents'," Linda said. "They believed that whatever the doctor said was the final word. But we're not like that. We go to the doctor, of course, and we have our regular screenings. But we listen to ourselves too. And we question the doctors. We get second opinions."

Linda found this attitude essential in caring for her son Leif, who had Down syndrome. Being his advocate included asking questions, taking notes, watching for errors. "It was like earning a degree in itself," said Linda. That was the only way they could feel assured that their son was getting the care he needed—not too little and not too much.

Eleven years later, this same proactive attitude is helping Linda to care for her own health needs as she grows older. Aware that her health depends largely on her own good habits, she makes time in her new retirement schedule for yoga and aerobics at the gym. She also plans to "destress" with meditation and hobbies like writing and painting. She and Clark stay socially active by volunteering with a community group that takes young people with disabilities skiing. But she doesn't want to get overbooked. Until recently, she needed time to visit her ninety-year-old mother, who lived at a memory-care facility until she died from Alzheimer's disease.

As for her own plans in old age, it's hard to say. But like many boomers, Linda's recent experience with her mother's prolonged illness and dependency has given her an even greater incentive to stay healthy as long as possible. She wants to build the mental, physical, and social reserves needed to keep living independently into her nineties.

In our conversation, I reminded Linda what another relative told me he would do if he were afflicted by the dementia that left his ninety-two-year-old father in a nursing home: he said he'd wait for a blizzard, head into the woods with a couple bottles of good red wine, enjoy drinking it, and then settle into a snowbank and go to sleep. "For us, I don't think that scenario is probable," she sighed.

Most boomers would agree with Linda. They won't choose the snow-drift; they want to grow old with independence and grace. And I predict that like women reading *Our Bodies, Ourselves*, they will want to arm themselves with knowledge about their options.

"IF I'D KNOWN I WAS GOING TO LIVE THIS LONG, I'D HAVE TAKEN BETTER CARE OF MYSELF"

That line may have earned laughs for composer Eubie Blake before he died in 1983. Baseball star Mickey Mantle repeated it later on. And country singer Merle Haggard wrote it into a song just before he died at age seventy-nine. But take note: these guys were all at least a generation older than the baby boomers with our longer life expectancy. For us, the joke may hit a little too close to home.

Here's the problem: the baby boom—defined as the seventy-eight million Americans born between 1946 to 1964—is expected to live about three years longer than their parents' generation did. We're benefiting, experts say, from growing up in a more prosperous economy with better education, better employment opportunities, medical advances, lower smoking rates, and better access to health care.

But we also have much higher rates of obesity-related disability and chronic illness than our parents' generation did at the same age. So unless the trend is reversed, many boomers may gain a few extra years only to spend them in poor health, disability, and dependency. The way out of this conundrum is for boomers to reverse course *now* by taking action to build the mental, physical, and social reserves needed to be healthy into old age.

The boomers' challenge is made clear in studies like the National Health and Nutrition Examination Survey (NHANES), a snapshot of self-reported health funded by the Centers for Disease Control and Prevention (CDC). In 2013, Dana King of West Virginia School of Medicine and colleagues published an analysis of the NHANES data in *JAMA Internal Medicine*.[5] They compared boomers aged forty-six to sixty-four between 2007 and 2010 to people who were the same age between 1988 and 1994 (see table 2.1).

The result? Only 13 percent of boomers rated their health as "excellent" while far more than twice as many—32 percent—of their parents' generation rated themselves that way at the same time of life.

The boomers also reported significantly higher rates of obesity-related chronic high blood pressure, diabetes, and high cholesterol. In addition, they had more limitations in their ability to do everyday functions, like walking up a flight of stairs or mowing the lawn; some 13 percent of the boomers said they had trouble with these tasks, compared to 9

Table 2.1. NHANES Analysis of Health Status, as Reported by Boomers and Their Parents' Generation

	Percent of Boomers' Parents Who Agreed (Surveyed 1988–1994)	Percent of Boomers Who Agreed (Surveyed 2007–2010)
I'm in excellent health	32	13
I'm obese	29	39
I exercise regularly	50	35
I have functional limitations in daily life	9	14
I need a walking device (such as a cane)	3	7
I've been diagnosed with diabetes	12	16
I'm taking medication for diabetes	6	11
I've been diagnosed with high cholesterol	34	74
I'm taking medication for high cholesterol	2	30
I've been diagnosed with high blood pressure	36	43
I'm taking medication for high blood pressure	23	35

percent of the older generation at the same age. About 7 percent of the boomers were using a cane or other device to get around, but only 3 percent of the parents' generation relied on such equipment.

Not all the news in Dr. King's analysis was bad, however. Boomers had less emphysema and fewer heart attacks than the earlier group— probably due to their lower rates of smoking.

But the NHANES report showed that the epidemic of obesity in our society is clearly taking its toll. About four in ten boomers were obese, compared with three in ten in the older generation. Lack of regular physical activity may be to blame. The analysis revealed that 35 percent of those middle-agers were getting moderate physical activity twelve times a month. That's far less than the 50 percent who reported doing so two decades earlier.

A longitudinal study of self-reported health status among four generations of Canadians (whose health habits are similar to Americans') revealed similar findings. Published in the health policy journal *Milbank Quarterly* in 2015, the study compared the health and habits of boomers to those slightly older. They found that the boomers were no healthier, despite their higher levels of education, and income, lower smoking rates, and greater access to health care, including immunizations and use of antibiotics for infectious disease. The researchers contended that such advantages among the boomers were "counterbalanced by adverse health factors such as increasing body mass index (i.e., being overweight and obese), resulting in no overall health improvement."[6]

What's the problem? Public health experts say our society's obesity epidemic is driven by lack of physical activity along with a notoriously poor diet. Intense marketing and easy access to calorie-rich, unhealthy foods are primary culprits. Also, we're spending more time in front of computer screens and televisions, and less time moving. Work life used to involve walking around offices, warehouses, and factories; now we're sitting at desks forty hours a week. Even our leisure hours have become less active. Instead of shopping on foot, we can order home delivery of nearly anything from online retailers. Why walk to the library when you can download books onto your iPhone or Kindle? You don't have to leave home to socialize; coffee klatches have been replaced by texting and Facebook chats.

There are pockets of hope—including slight increases in recreational exercise among some portions of the boomer population (think aerobic dance classes or weightlifting). A 2015 CDC report showed that the percentage of Americans aged fifty-five to sixty-four who got enough weekly aerobic or muscle-strengthening activity to meet federal guidelines rose from about 13 percent during 2002 to 2003 to about 16 percent during 2012 to 2013.[7] (These guidelines call for at least 150 minutes a week of moderate-intensity exercise or seventy-five minutes a week of vigorous intensive aerobic exercise, or an equal equivalent combination of both. Also, muscle strengthening should happen two days a week or more.)

Still, evidence continues to show increases in boomers with obesity-related chronic disease. Moreover, research reveals that obesity-linked illness takes a disproportionate toll among racial minorities and people in lower socioeconomic levels. Those with lower levels of education and income are much more likely to be obese and suffer the consequent poor health effects. Over time, health-related disparities related to socioeconomic status have been increasing for all age groups.

Also worrisome is the tremendous increase in drug treatment for these obesity-related conditions. This raises the question of whether boomers have become too reliant on medication. The NHANES data showed, for example, that drug use for high cholesterol was *twenty times higher* among the boomers than for the previous generation. Treatment for high blood pressure went from 23 percent to 35 percent, and treatment for diabetes nearly doubled.

"The drugs are supposed to be used *in addition* to a healthy lifestyle, not instead of it," Dr. King told the press when his analysis was published.[8] Of course, some of the drugs boomers reported taking for these conditions were not widely available two decades previously. But the question remains: are such drug treatments masking symptoms of health problems that could actually be "cured" with lifestyle changes?

"Medication use has definitely increased, so we are propping ourselves up on our canes and our medicines," said Dr. King. "We are becoming overdependent on medications and surgical solutions rather than creating our own good health."

If you find Dr. King's words a little scary, take heart: he also told the press that people aged fifty to seventy still have time to "turn back the clock," and I agree. The challenge is to do what Eubie Blake, Mickey Mantle, and Merle Haggard wished they had done sooner—*take better care of themselves.*

BUT WHAT KIND OF CARE—AND HOW MUCH—DO WE NEED?

These are important questions in today's health care system—where a passive approach can too easily result in unintended harm. The alternative is to take an *active* approach, one that puts you in charge of your health and health care. That's what you'll need to build the mental, physical, and social reserves needed to live well into old age.

People on the passive end of the spectrum tend to ignore their health until something goes wrong. Then they rely on physicians and other health care providers to determine what tests and care they need, no questions asked. They may be curious about their health, but they lack confidence in their own ability to seek health information and improve their well-being through changes in physical activity, diet, stress reduction, and so on.

In my experience as a physician and person who's also aging, this passive attitude seems more common among older generations—people who came of age before "Question Authority" became a T-shirt slogan. That was also before the public had access to good health information through the media and Internet. As *Our Bodies, Ourselves* demonstrated, knowledge is power. So until patients were able to obtain the information needed, control over health care decisions rested squarely in the doctor's court.

At the other end of the spectrum are health activists. These are people who see their doctors as important advisors for staying well. They look to their health care providers for recommendations on prevention, screening, and treatment. They engage in proactive decision making with their doctors by asking questions, weighing the pros and cons based on their own values, and communicating their choices. They realize that they are building a foundation of healthy reserves for future use. And they understand that, ultimately, the real work happens not at the clinic, but at home on a daily basis as a result of their own attitudes and habits.

Most people fall somewhere in the middle of this range. Studies have shown that many Americans are dissatisfied with their level of involvement in health care decisions and would like to be more engaged. The level of participation desired may differ by age, education level, and race or ethnicity—with younger and more educated people being the most likely to prefer an active role. However, older, minority, and low-literacy individuals also want to become more involved in their treatment decisions. These people tend to seek an active role when they feel knowledgeable and have confidence in their ability to understand, manage, and communicate health concerns.

For those who want to take an active role, I believe it's well worth the necessary time and effort, because it tends to result in having a longer, healthier, more satisfying life.

AVOIDING OVERDIAGNOSIS AND OVERTREATMENT

Being a health care activist can also protect you from American medicine's troubling propensity to offer too many blood tests, assessments, scans, procedures, surgeries, and prescription drugs. In a society where we tend to believe that more of anything is better, it may be hard to understand how more attention and services from health care professionals could be a bad thing. But here's the problem: sometimes a test or a diagnosis is just the first step in a cascade of events that leads to unnecessary care and even harm. Journalist and health policy expert Shannon Brownlee describes it as "a therapeutic cascade—you start to tumble downstream to more and more invasive testing, and possibly even treatment for things that should be left well enough alone."[9]

The alternative is to seek what a colleague of mine calls "Goldilocks care" or "high-value care"—it's not too little and not too much. It's just right because it balances how much a test or treatment could help you against how much it could harm you.

Appropriate screening and lifestyle changes are high value because they are low risk and help prevent you from getting sick and needing harmful or expensive medical care. Low-value care is just the opposite. It includes tests and procedures that are not right for your level of risk, result in too many false alarms, waste your time and money, and unnecessarily expose you to hazards like radiation or unnecessary surgeries.

In 2012, the American Board of Internal Medicine joined forces with *Consumer Reports* to start a campaign called Choosing Wisely, which promotes conversations among physicians and their patients to eliminate low-value tests and treatments. The campaign's patient website (www.consumerhealthchoices.org) provides a terrific guide for patients who want to have such conversations with their doctors.

Problems of overdiagnosis and overtreatment are particularly concerning for older people because they typically have more contacts with the health care system. Trouble can range from increased cost and inconvenience to higher risk of adverse effects from unnecessary, unwarranted drugs or surgeries that are not likely to provide benefit. For elderly people who generally have more sensitivity to medications, stress, and medical intervention, this cascade of events can make the treatment more dangerous than the issue the doctor is trying to address.

Overdiagnosis often stems from a conventional belief that it's good to catch diseases early, and that's certainly true for some conditions, such as colon cancer and certain kinds of breast cancer. But often, in our overzealousness to provide early detection, we can actually cause more harm than good.

H. Gilbert Welch, a professor of medicine at the Dartmouth Institute for Health Policy and Clinical Practice, has done extensive research and education to help people understand how too much care can hurt. Harm can occur "when doctors make diagnoses in individuals who are not destined to ever develop symptoms or die from the condition diagnosed," he said.[10]

The classic example is the widespread use of prostate cancer screening, which began in the early 1990s following the development of prostate-specific antigen (PSA) blood tests. PSA is a protein that's produced by the prostate gland and is often elevated in men who have prostate cancer. But the PSA test has many drawbacks. For example, some tumors found through PSA testing grow so slowly that they are unlikely to ever become life threatening. Treating them with surgery or radiation, however, can cause harmful side effects such as urinary incontinence, problems with bowel function, and trouble having erections. Because of these limitations, most medical societies and the U.S. Preventive Services Task Force have stopped recommending PSA testing in recent years—but not before more than a million men were unnecessarily treated for a cancer that was never going to bother them, Dr. Welch explained. "More than a third of these men suffered serious effects," he added.[11]

Overdiagnosis can occur as a result of routine breast cancer screening as well. While mammograms can detect dangerous forms of invasive breast cancer early, this technology has limits, and using it too frequently to screen large populations of healthy women is problematic. Surprisingly, Dr. Welch's research has shown that screening mammography has had little impact on breast cancer death rates.[12] But it has resulted in large populations of women "receiving some combination of surgery, chemotherapy and/or radiation, when, in fact, that cancer was not destined to cause symptoms—a lump you can feel—or be life-threatening," he writes.[13] One example is ductal carcinoma in situ (DCIS), a common breast disease that is often treated like cancer but rarely becomes invasive. Finding it more frequently via screening mammography is resulting in higher rates of diagnosis and treatment, but it's not improving health outcomes for women in screening programs.

Experts believe we need clearer recognition that breast cancer screening methods don't work equally well for all women or for all different kinds of breast disease. Therefore, to avoid overdiagnosis and overtreatment, health care needs to offer a more personalized approach, providing screening based on women's individual risk factors. These include family history of breast cancer, personal health history, and a person's genetic risk. By doing so, we can avoid the harms of unnecessary radiation exposure and unneeded treatment.

Our evolving understanding of breast cancer has caused the medical establishment to revisit breast cancer screening guidelines in recent years. For example, in 2015 the American Cancer Society and the U.S. Preventive Services Task Force (USPSTF) changed their screening recommendations to make screening mammography less frequent for younger women.[14] Also, the USPSTF has stated that there's insufficient evidence to support breast cancer screening for women seventy-five and older.[15]

I'm certain our understanding of cancer screening will improve based on ongoing research. In the meantime, discussion of breast cancer screening guidelines typically evokes strong opinions from people concerned about women's health, and understandably so. Breast cancer is the second most common cause of cancer death in the United States. So it makes sense for providers, researchers, health policy makers—and patients themselves—to pay careful attention to prevention and screening efforts.

For this and all types of tests, being an activated patient means talking with your doctor about your individual risks and determining a plan that fits your personal risk profile, medical history, and values. This is true in screening for many kinds of illness, including mammography for breast cancer, routine EKGs or stress tests for heart disease, or assessment for Alzheimer's disease. Being an activated ager requires learning the benefits, limitations, and potential harms of tests and treatments. And perhaps most importantly, if you notice symptoms or changes in your body that concern you, you should call a trusted health care professional who can answer your questions and help you decide next steps.

THE TROUBLE WITH HIGH-END IMAGING

Among modern medicine's most beneficial advances is the use of high-end imaging to see inside the body and detect diseases that need treatment. Examples include various forms of radiology, such as computed tomography (CT) scans, positron emissions tomography (PET) scans, and magnetic resonance imaging (MRI). While such advances have been a tremendous boon—especially when looking for problems such as lethal but treatable cancerous tumors—this technology also comes with risks that we need to manage. CT scans, for example, can involve a high level of exposure to radiation, which can increase your risk for cancer. High-end imaging may also result in finding (and treating) harmless abnormalities while looking for more dire problems. Unless doctors can discern which findings are worth treating and which should be left alone, patients may undergo potentially harmful procedures to remove noncancerous and slow-growing tumors or cysts (sometimes called "incidentalomas") unlikely to cause illness or death.

The challenge is to use advanced imaging technology wisely. When imaging is considered, doctors and patients need to determine if the scan is really necessary. Questions to ask may include these:

- Can the test in question provide new information that will make a difference in the patient's care?
- What are the risks and benefits of treatment that might result from this information?
- Will the information discovered through this test change our plan for care?

As we'll explore in chapter 8, these are particularly important questions for people late in life, when frailty might preclude surgery no matter what the finding, or a cancer is so slow-growing that the patient is more likely to die from other causes first. In situations like these, avoiding imaging might also prevent the patient from having to undergo the stress, pain, and possible complications of surgery.

Caution is advised for younger, healthier people as well—especially when considering imaging for a condition that might be resolved by noninvasive means. Low back pain is a good example. When I did my medical training in the 1970s, the causes of common back pain were not as well understood as they are currently. We were taught to consider imaging early to determine if people needed back surgery. Since the 1990s, however, medical experts have learned that jumping to these solutions too soon is unwise and may even lead to unnecessary surgery that doesn't address the primary causes of the pain—issues such as lack of exercise, poor posture while working all day at a computer, or other job-related physical and emotional stresses. There's a better recognition that back pain may be just part of the human condition. We now know that nearly all cases of acute back pain get better within a few days or weeks. And for those that don't, exercise such as yoga is remarkably effective. There is a certain small portion of people who need surgery if spinal nerves or the spinal cord itself are involved, and for these people, surgery typically should be considered a last resort.

Getting to the root causes of back pain can be a challenge, particularly if patients (and their doctors) misunderstand the implications of "abnormalities" seen on x-ray images—problems such as degenerated or protruding spinal discs. University of Washington neuroradiologist Jeffrey Jarvik is addressing this challenge based on an important study he published in 2001 using MRI images of the low back from 148 Veterans' Administration patients *without* back pain. His team found, for example, that 91 percent of these MRIs showed degenerated spinal discs, more than 64 percent showed bulging discs, and 32 percent showed disc protrusion. But none of these patients were reporting pain as a result of these problems.[16]

As Dr. Welch explained to NPR, "Almost all of us harbor meniscal (cartilage) tears in our knees, whether or not we have knee pain. We have discs popping out of our backs whether or not we have a back pain. So the problem is, we're identifying so many 'abnormalities' in normal people."[17] This puts pressure on patients and doctors to seek complex, invasive, or risky surgical solutions when a simpler approach might be wiser.

So now Dr. Jarvik is leading a study set at Group Health Cooperative and elsewhere to see if providing doctors with this information as context on back-pain patients' radiology reports can influence their physicians' approach to subsequent treatment. For instance, will such reports decrease the prevalence of additional testing, narcotic prescriptions, or referrals to back surgery? Can we avoid overtreatment simply by giving physicians and their patients more information about the appearance of a normal, pain-free back? Dr. Jarvik's team hopes to find out.

TOO MANY PILLS, BUT NO QUICK FIXES

Meanwhile, the problems of overtreatment are widespread. In a study published in *JAMA Internal Medicine* in 2013, Harvard researcher John N. Mafi and colleagues found problems nationwide among physicians who don't follow approved back-pain treatment guidelines such as avoiding high-end imaging, using nonopioid painkillers, and referring patients to physical therapy.[18] Their survey of nearly twenty-four thousand visits over twelve years, showed advanced imaging rose by 60 percent, use of narcotics increased by 51 percent, and referrals to other physicians, often for surgery, doubled. Findings like these should motivate the activist ager to raise a red flag whenever they believe their doctor might be ordering too many drugs, tests, or procedures.

The harm to our society from overprescribing opioids—a type of narcotic painkiller such as Vicodin or OxyContin—can't be overstated. More than a quarter million people lost their lives to opioid overdoses in the United States between 2000 and 2015.[19] Overuse of opioids for noncancer chronic pain is the worst iatrogenic (medically caused) epidemic of our lifetime, according to my colleague Michael Von Korff, ScD, a health services researcher at Group Health Research Institute.[20] Some thirty thousand people in the United States died from opioid overdose in 2015 alone.[21]

But opioids are certainly not the only class of drugs that have been overprescribed. Historic examples include the use of estrogen replacement (hormone therapy), which was commonly recommended to women for decades not just to treat bothersome symptoms of menopause but to reduce risks related to vascular diseases, breast cancer, and osteoporosis. Once the Women's Health Initiative found in 2002 that estrogen replacement therapy actually *increased* women's risk of vascular disease and certain cancers,[22] its use tapered off. But these drugs are still routinely given for other uses, such as risk of fractures. Women who take them for such purposes should be aware of the cancer and cardiovascular risks involved.

Overuse of antibiotics has long been a problem as well. Often, patients ask their doctors for antibacterial antibiotics such as penicillin, thinking they will provide quick relief for colds or other upper respiratory infections such as a sinus infection, bronchitis, or a sore throat. But such illnesses are almost always caused by viruses, which don't respond to antibiotics. Taking antibiotics inappropriately won't help with your symptoms, but can lead to the development of antibiotic-resistant bacteria, which are difficult to treat.

Whether for pain, sleep, digestion, heart problems, anxiety, depression, incontinence, osteoporosis, or any other health concern—the list of drugs a person takes often grows longer with age, and not always with a good result. As I mentioned earlier related to the NHANES study, prescriptions for chronic health problems such as high blood pressure, high cholesterol, and diabetes are on the rise. Part of this is related to a broadening of guidelines, resulting in more people being considered at risk for cardiovascular disease. There's no doubt that such drugs have benefited millions of people by averting heart attacks and strokes. But when guidelines are broadened, the newly created "patients" may get less benefit from the drug than the original target population, yet the potential harm from side effects is just as great. Let me give you an example. Some experts have recommended that the threshold for prescribing blood-pressure-lowering medication be lowered from a systolic pressure of 130 mmHg to 120 mmHg. Those whose blood pressure hovers around 140 will clearly get more benefit from the medication than those with a usual blood pressure of, say, 125. But they may both face the same level of risk for possible side effects from the drug, such as fatigue or dizziness.

As a patient, it is hard to stay abreast of such changes in prescription guidelines. You rely on your doctor for such information about the drugs you may be prescribed, and rightly so. But as an activated ager, it's good to know about this general phenomenon toward broadening guidelines to include more and more people who are at lower risk for the diseases the drugs are meant to treat. You'll want to talk with your doctor about a recommended drug's benefits and the risks for you as an individual. And you may also want to ask whether changes such as exercising more or eating a healthier diet might make the drug unnecessary for you altogether.

And no matter what medications you're taking, you'll want to recognize that medication is just one limited way to take care of your health; it's no substitute for healthy habits that can lead to better overall health and quality of life. Consider the positive impact that exercise and a healthy diet can have on a whole range of health issues, including postponing dementia and preventing mood disorders, osteoporosis, diabetes, joint and back pain, sleeping problems, cancer, general weakness, fatigue, and more. If you are diagnosed with hypertension, atherosclerosis, or some other forms of cardiovascular disease, it would be a shame for you to forgo exercise and dietary changes because you felt that your blood pressure medication or anticholesterol drugs had you covered. By relying only on drugs and forgoing lifestyle changes, you'd be missing out on a whole host of ways to make your life better.

We'll discuss many drug treatments in chapter 6 as we explore ways to build physical reserve, but here are two key points for activist agers to consider when discussing new drug recommendations with their health care teams:

1. *The newest drug is not necessarily the best.* Drug companies have strong financial incentives to introduce new drugs, especially when there's no equivalent generic version that can be sold as a substitute at a much lower price. As Dr. Welch explains, "The easiest way for pharmaceutical companies to make money isn't to build a better drug or device—it's to expand the market for existing drugs and devices by expanding the indication to include more patients."[23] Consequently, drug marketers encourage consumers to "ask your doctor" about "new and improved" versions of medications for common health problems. But new potential side effects may not appear until after the drug has been used for a while among large, general populations. So I generally like to wait five or more years before changing my recommendations from a tried-and-true medication to a new one. This allows enough time to ensure that the new medication is truly safe, effective, and worth any extra cost. For many common health conditions such as high blood pressure, diabetes, and high cholesterol, there are actually plenty of good drugs available that have stood the test of time; in these cases, there's little reason to encourage my patients to become early adopters of a relatively new,

unproven product. And over the years, this approach has allowed me to help my patients avoid side effects that were not discovered until some years after a drug had been on the market.

2. *All drug treatments have possible side effects.* Whenever you start a new medication, talk to your doctor about what to expect. Then see if you notice any of these or other effects. Problems with balance, dizziness, or feeling faint are particularly significant because of the risk that you could fall and seriously injure yourself. Symptoms of sleepiness, loss of appetite, confusion, or trouble thinking are also important to report. Besides interfering with your quality of life, such symptoms may lead to an inappropriate diagnosis of Alzheimer's or other brain disease. Many drugs commonly prescribed for issues such as hay fever, incontinence, anxiety, depression, and insomnia cause problems with thinking and behavior. So if you're on a new medication and experience such trouble, bring it to your doctor's attention right away. Ask if there are alternative medications or changes in lifestyle that you might try for managing your condition.

COULD EXERCISE BE THE MAGIC BULLET?

When I consider the many health problems treated—and often over-treated—with medication and procedures, I see a common theme: Western medicine's attempt to sell quick fixes—that is, medical solutions to complex problems that might be better addressed with lifestyle changes related to exercise.

It's probably human nature to wish for the "magic bullet," the pill or other treatment to solve the problem without having to change ingrained patterns of physical inactivity. And yet the science is clear on two important points: (1) all treatments have related adverse effects, and (2) regular exercise can turn the tide on chronic conditions that put us at risk for cardiovascular disease, cancer, depression, and more. Whether it's bicycling for cardiovascular health, yoga to prevent back pain, or walking to postpone symptoms of Alzheimer's disease, evidence shows that routine exercise, combined with a healthy diet, can reduce or eliminate our need for various medications and medical interventions.

While avoiding medication can be strong motivation to start exercising regularly, there are, of course, many other reasons. Consider the significance of growing older with the capacity to keep moving well, thinking clearly, and avoiding falls and mishaps. By building and maintaining your endurance, strength, coordination, balance, and energy through exercise, you'll have a better chance of avoiding disability. You may increase your time available for travel, getting out in nature, living independently, being a vital part of your family and community—in other words, doing what you want to do.

I'm reminded of Mike Evans, a family medicine doctor and researcher from the University of Toronto whose nine-minute YouTube video "23 and 1/2 Hours: What Is the Single Best Thing We Can Do for Our Health?" has been seen by millions of viewers.[24] His message is so simple and yet so powerful: spend just thirty minutes a day on exercise to vastly improve the quality of every other minute of your life. His quick review of the scientific evidence showing benefits among patients at risk for arthritis, dementia, diabetes, hip fracture, anxiety, depression—and yes, even death—supports his thesis: exercise is by far the best medicine you can take to prevent problems such as these from ruining your health.

I have seen this logic work wonders for patients, especially those with high blood pressure (hypertension), high cholesterol, and diabetes. All three of these conditions put people at much higher risk for heart disease and early death. But once a person is motivated to change their habits over the long term, and gets the support needed to do so, they can make changes that may alter the course of their lives. Rather than spending their last decades feeling too sick and disabled to pursue dreams for their retirement years, they have the strength and energy to fully participate in life.

That's not to say that change comes easily. If that were true, I think we would see far fewer people suffering from obesity-related illnesses. But change *is* possible for those who are motivated and have the support they need to make it happen. Boomers in the United States have seen this demonstrated in their lifetime on a large scale as we turned the tide on our national epidemic of tobacco addiction. Smoking rates among American adults have dropped from 42 percent in 1965 to 17 percent in 2014. Granted, there are differences in the problems of smoking and the causes of obesity. But for the individuals suffering the effects of either problem, making healthy changes usually requires significant amounts of motivation and support. And sometimes that motivation and support comes on the heels of a health crisis.

CHANGE OF HEART, CHANGE OF MIND

When Kirk Williamson was laid off from his job as a communications consultant in June 2015, he figured it was a good time to start making other changes as well. He bought a bicycle and was planning to get in shape. But after thirty years of sedentary living, the challenge seemed daunting. At age sixty-six, he was more than one hundred pounds overweight and had high blood pressure. Climbing stairs or walking a few city blocks was difficult. In September, when he and his daughter tried to hike up Badger Mountain—a popular overlook near his hometown of Kennewick, Washington—Kirk had to turn back.

"I was feeling pretty fatalistic," he said later. "I thought, 'If I'm lucky, I'll have the Big One and then it won't matter.' . . . I'm pretty sure my family was getting tired of hearing me talk about what kind of funeral service I wanted, but that's what was going on."[25]

Kirk didn't have that major heart attack, however. Instead, his doctor found an irregular heartbeat while treating him for an unrelated problem that fall. Not surprisingly, he had some follow-up tests, and eventually an angiogram showed that all four major arteries in his heart were clogged 80 to 90 percent. The situation was life threatening. He would need bypass surgery right away.

The surgery successfully cleared away the blockages. Afterward, Kirk went through months of cardiovascular rehabilitation—treatment that strengthened not only his heart but also his mind as he developed a new, proactive attitude toward caring for his health.

In truth, Kirk had always considered himself an activist—especially when it came to things like government and social responsibility. He'd been a leader in local politics and service clubs like the Kiwanis.

And he took his relationship to health care seriously as well. "I would talk to my doctor about my blood pressure medication and whether I should have a PSA test," he explained. "I got my colonoscopy on time. So I was engaged at that level. I just wasn't engaged at the get-off-your-butt-and-walk-around-the-block level, or the don't-eat-that-hamburger level."

As a child of the 1960s, Kirk had great faith in science and technology. "I remember Sputnik and the space race and all those incredible technological advances," he said. His trust carried over into health care. "I figured, whatever the problem is, they will find a way to fix it."

But beyond medication, Kirk found no simple fix for his high blood pressure and obesity. As his weight increased over the years, so did his frustration with exercise and dieting. Occasionally he would consider joining a health club. "But then I thought, I'm not going in there with a bunch of women in Spandex," he said.

He also thought about bariatric surgery, but that seemed too extreme. Besides, he knew a friend who had the surgery, lost weight, and then gained it right back.

Kirk understood what he needed to do. "It was just, how do you start eating better and exercising more—and then make it stick? I just *could not* do that. Then I felt guilty because I couldn't. And you know where guilt leads you? It makes you want to eat!" he laughs with humility.

After his heart surgery in early November, however, Kirk's relationship to the problem changed. It wasn't like he suddenly "saw the light" and was able to do everything right. In fact, he admits that after the operation, he felt he was simply "going through the motions" his rehab required. But I believe his willingness to give himself over to the rehab process allowed an important transformation to occur.

In early January 2016, after several weeks of rest at home, Kirk started going to a cardiac rehabilitation program—a specialized gym where he worked out several days a week under the watchful eye of a cardiac nurse and exercise therapist. With that support, he started to experience and track small, incremental changes that built his confidence in himself to succeed with his new habits over time. This is something health-behavior experts refer to as building "self-efficacy." You see that the small steps you're taking are helping you to achieve the result you want. And that evidence convinces you to keep going—which leads to a cycle of further success.

"At first, it was gruesome," Kirk jokes. "I could barely stand up on the treadmill, much less walk on it." But with each session, he increased his time and intensity on the facility's various exercise machines.

The staff convinced Kirk that it was safe to push himself, despite his recent surgery. They also encouraged him gradually to pick up the pace. "I'd be practically sweating blood, and here would come Ashley to say, 'How hard are you working up there?' I'd say, 'Um . . . let me turn this thing up a bit.'"

Kirk changed his diet, eating many of the same foods he's always loved but in much smaller portions. He also kept track each day of his weight, his blood pressure, and his physical activity. "After a while, it started to sink in that I was having some success," he said.

For one, he was able to go from four blood-pressure medications to just two. Moreover, by March, he had lost about forty pounds and was feeling well enough to take a long-anticipated vacation to the Southwest.

"My wife and I had a great time," he said. Their shared interest in technology led them to tour Biosphere 2, an earth systems research facility near Tucson. "It's got lots of steps and I never would have made it a year ago," he said. "This time, I was up and down all over the place."

I've seen many other patients have this kind of success as well. Whether they're dealing with smoking cessation, alcohol problems, overeating, or changing their patterns of physical activity, behavior change can be very challenging. But based on what I was taught decades ago, the payoff is often far greater than I would ever have expected. And because it can be so difficult *and* rewarding, getting support from coaches, teachers, counselors, or sponsors in a structured program is often well worthwhile.

For some people, that assistance comes from organizations like Weight Watchers, Alcoholics Anonymous, or a phone-based stop-smoking quit line. Many people also find online applications helpful. Kirk's support for exercise came from his cardiac rehab team. But people also find motivation through senior centers, local gyms, or the YMCA. A personal trainer or coach can also be a great help, if you can afford it. The point is, if you're having trouble making important changes and you're going it alone, consider reaching out to others for help.

By April, Kirk had started to eye Badger Mountain again. That's the trail he had tried—and failed—to climb with his daughter before his operation. But he had lost fifty-five pounds since then. He asked the rehab nurse if she thought the trail was safe for him, and she gave him a thumbs-up.

So on April 7—150 days after his surgery—Kirk hiked the Skyline Trail, which gains 796 vertical feet in just under two miles. He returned to the mountain a week later with his eleven-year-old grandson, Will, and hiked it again. Since then, he's tried other trails around the legendary mountain, including the Canyon Trail, which is shorter but much steeper. He can't seem to get enough of its fifty-mile views.

Not yet ready to retire, Kirk is working on his second career. He has a new part-time job, taking guests from a Columbia River steamboat company on tours of area wineries. He's also applying to become a substitute elementary school teacher. Inspiration came the day his Kiwanis Club accompanied a bunch of third graders on a tour of historic Kennewick. "A year ago, I wasn't sure I could walk that far. But I did it," he said, "and I really enjoyed being with the kids."

On days he doesn't hike, he rides his bike along a Columbia River trail. If the weather's bad, he walks at an indoor shopping mall. He said he might even join a gym, Spandex be damned.

"I have a whole different attitude about things," he said. "I feel like I did when I was forty. And I've got energy. I wake up in the morning and I'm interested in what's going on in the world."

HAVING IT YOUR WAY: SHARED DECISION MAKING

Being proactive about your health can range from taking charge of your own everyday health habits—as Kirk did—to being more engaged with your health care team in care decisions. Fortunately, American health care providers appear to be moving toward becoming more "patient centered"—that is, giving patients a greater role in determining what tests, treatments, and care plans to pursue for various health conditions. When doctors do this, they can be more assured that the care they provide is aligned with patients' values.

One sign that patient-centered care is catching on is health care systems' increasing adoption of "shared decision making"—where patients work closely with their doctors or other care providers to consider the pros and cons of various treatment decisions.

Say, for example, you have serious knee pain that's slowing you down. You think knee replacement might be a possibility for you, but you're not sure. Maybe there are other options, such as continuing to treat the pain with over-the-counter pain relievers. Gentle exercise also seems to help. Plus, your doctor has told you weight loss would make a difference. But your best friend, who has a new knee, is encouraging you to get the surgery soon: "Get it over with. You'll feel so much better in no time." Meanwhile your neighbor warns, "Don't do it! The recovery is awful! And there could be complications!"

Shared decision making helps to sort through this kind of chatter. Patients find it particularly helpful as they age and are faced with increasingly more treatment choices. Shared decision making can be especially important when (1) there is more than one reasonable option, (2) no single option has a clear advantage, and (3) the possible benefits and harms of each option affect patients differently.

In shared decision making, the patient is typically directed to a "decision aid"—a video, brochure, or website that's easy to understand and provides unbiased clinical evidence about the care in question. Sometimes patients are put in touch with a trained coach or "navigator" as well. The information they receive is designed to be objective, balancing risks and expected outcomes with the patient's preferences and values. The goal is to help patients become more knowledgeable about their health condition and treatment options, to decide which risks and benefits are most important to them, and to envision how different options would affect their daily lives.

Shared decision making is often used when considering treatment for conditions providers call "preference sensitive"—things like prostate cancer screening, bariatric surgery for obesity, breast reconstruction following a mastectomy, and surgery for uterine fibroids or prostate conditions. For conditions like these, there's not enough scientific evidence to provide a clear-cut yes or no recommendation for all individuals. That's why the patient's preferences and values need to be a big part of the decision. Shared decision-making processes are designed to make sure the deliberation between doctors and patients happens. Decision aids are also being developed to help people with terminal conditions make decisions about withdrawing life-sustaining treatment.

Interest in shared decision making has grown in recent years for many reasons.

One, it's superior to the way many people have made health care decisions in the past—by listening to just one doctor who may or may not have biases based on a variety of influences. Progress toward health-reform measures in recent years are helping to eliminate profit motives that might encourage physicians in fee-for-service systems to encourage more treatment than necessary. But it can be difficult for even the most objective doctor to describe all the risks and benefits of a potential treatment for any given patient—especially when there's not enough scientific evidence to support one position or the other. Studies have shown that doctors spend more time explaining the advantages of a procedure than they do outlining the disadvantages.

Also, like any other profession, doctors are highly influenced by their peers and the communities in which they practice. Studies conducted by Dartmouth Medical School and others have revealed that a patient's geographical location may influence which care options they receive. Researchers found, for example, that patients got more surgery for certain conditions per capita in places like Miami than, say, Seattle, where medicine is practiced more conservatively. It wasn't that there were more arthritic hips among elderly people in Miami; rather, there were more surgeons in Miami promoting the operation to their patients.

Interestingly, research has revealed differences like these on a local level too. For example, when doctors at Group Health Cooperative compared their own surgery rates, they found unwarranted differentiation within their own ranks. In other words, doctors at various Group Health clinics around Seattle were practicing differently than doctors at other Group Health clinics—despite all working within the same regional health care system. This revelation motivated the group to become more interested in shared decision making because they understood that it shouldn't matter which neighborhood you live in; the individual patient's history and values should be a more significant factor in the options he or she receives. Now, when a patient is a candidate for shared decision making, doctors get a prompt from the electronic medical record to direct the patient to a decision aid that can help them better understand their condition and choices. Then they can have an informed conversation with the doctor about which way to go. Since starting its program in 2009, Group Health has distributed more shared decision-making aids than any other health care system worldwide.[26]

Reactions to shared decision-making programs have been positive. In 2011, a survey of 2,200 Group Health patients showed that 41 percent found the program extremely important, half found it very important, and 9 percent found it somewhat important.[27] Another study showed that people who engage in shared decision making better understand the risks and benefits of their care and are more likely to follow the treatment plan they agree upon with their doctor, which can lead to better health.[28]

In addition, shared decision making appears to be making a dent in the nation's epidemic of overtreatment and medical harm. Research shows that patients who participate in such processes typically choose less invasive, less complex forms of care. We found this to be true for joint replacement surgery at Group Health. In a study of 9,500 patients published in *Health Affairs* in 2012, Group Health Research Institute's Dr. David Arterburn showed that after establishing a program to provide patients with evidence-based information videos, the system had 26 percent fewer hip replacements, 38 percent fewer knee replacements, and a 12 percent to 21 percent reduction in costs for those patients over six months.[29]

The Group Health study was limited in that it reported just six months of data. Also, it looked only at hip and knee surgeries even though the program was distributing aids on a dozen topics. But many people involved in the initiative reported that it caused a shift in our doctors' awareness of patients' preferences and concerns. In other words, the culture of our organization had become more patient centered.

Here's an example: Wayne Grytting, sixty-eight, predicted that his Group Health doctor was going to recommend knee surgery for him when he showed up at the clinic complaining about the pain. On a scale of one to ten, with ten being the worst, Wayne told the doctor his knee pain was a seven. He said, "It was enough to keep me out of hiking, out of biking," two activities the writer and retired teacher dearly enjoys.[30]

But Wayne didn't want surgery if he could avoid it. So they talked about other options such as weight loss and doing physical therapy. If Wayne thought these options were worth trying, the doctor told him there was a significant chance he could make the pain dissipate without surgery.

"As I started doing the workouts every day—the stretches and the knee strengthening exercises—the pain started going away," Wayne remembered. Encouraged, he got back on his bicycle, and pretty soon the pain had completely disappeared.

Weight loss also helped. "I was carrying a bag of kitty litter up our stairs and I realized, my goodness, that's the weight I've taken off," Wayne said. Today, "I couldn't tell you which knee I had problems in."

And what if Wayne had chosen to just go ahead with the surgery? Within the culture of shared decision making, that would also be a success, as long as the patient's choice reflected his or her own values and best chances for a positive outcome.

As research has shown, the process of shared decision making can also benefit patients by helping them gauge their expectations. This may be especially true when self-care is needed to prepare for or recover from surgery, for example, or to manage a chronic condition.

That's how it's been for Wendy Townsend, a seventy-three-year-old yoga instructor with osteoarthritis who is anticipating a second hip replacement. In discussions with her Group Health surgeon about the procedure, "He says we'll do it when I'm ready," Wendy explained.[31]

She and her doctor agree that surgery is the right choice, in part because she did well with recovery from her first hip replacement when she was sixty. True, she's older now, but she has no other health problems, so a good outcome is expected with this upcoming surgery as well.

Wendy's doctor knows what's important to her—that she wants to keep teaching, traveling, taking daily walks with her friends, seeing her daughter and grandsons frequently. With goals like these, she'll have lots of motivation to do the rehabilitation exercises after surgery, and that also sets her up for a positive result. The doctor has encouraged her to stay as active as possible between now and the surgery, despite the pain she sometimes experiences. So she has added swimming to her weekly routine of yoga classes and walking. Doing so helps to ensure that she's feeling strong and healthy when she decides the time is right to schedule the operation.

I know as a practicing physician and researcher that most doctors inherently want to provide care that serves their patients' needs, desires, and values. I also know that many doctors have a natural bias toward action, to use the treatments and procedures we've been trained to use. In shared decision making, our work is to balance those two sets of goals to help create the best outcome for those we serve. As a patient, you can do your part by learning all you can about your care options and communicating your preferences and values to your doctor. That way, you'll be working as a team to keep you healthy as the years go by.

Ultimately, of course, good health depends on so much more than the conversations and activities that happen between doctors and patients. As people like Evangeline Shuler, Marcus Aquino, Kirk Williamson, and others have shown us, it depends on individuals taking action on their own behalf to build and maintain the resources needed for resilient aging. And as we'll learn in the next chapter, it also takes an acceptance of the changes that aging inevitably brings.

3

ACCEPTANCE

Discovering Aging on Its Own Terms

My longtime friend and colleague Meredith Pfanschmidt likes to walk the paved track around Seattle's Green Lake rain or shine, two or three times a week. Sometimes she does it alone, listening to NPR podcasts. More often she arranges to meet a friend for the 2.8-mile stroll. On this bright June morning, she pauses on the west shore where logs float amid luminous green lily pads.

"See the turtles sunning themselves?" she asks, pointing at the logs. "They're always there."[1]

Since retiring at age sixty-seven, Meredith has plenty of time to notice such wonders. Except for that precious period when her son was little, she figures this may be the most satisfying part of her life.

"I have more perspective," she says. "Maybe it's because I worked with older patients for so many years, or maybe it's just part of growing older myself—but I realize that my life could be over in a minute."

The thought doesn't seem to frighten her. Instead, it reminds her to enjoy each day as it comes. If the weather's nice, she might spend a whole afternoon in her yard, reading a novel or digging in her garden. If she's running errands and gets caught in traffic, she relaxes. There are no job-related appointments to keep. When a friend suggests they celebrate Meredith's seventieth birthday by venturing out of state to walk a half marathon, she figures, why not? Exercise, friendship, and travel are all top priorities for her right now.

I'm thrilled to see Meredith embrace her retirement in this way—especially after watching her juggle the demands of a career, single parenthood, and caring for her disabled brother, who recently died. She's still got obligations. She volunteers for a pet shelter and a hospice organization. Just taking care of the house where she raised her son is a chore. But she approaches her days with acceptance that life is finite, and this approach makes her happy.

HOW ACCEPTANCE HELPS HAPPINESS GROW

I've lately noticed more of my baby-boom peers taking the same stance Meredith has, and I'm glad. Such acceptance—when combined with knowledge about aging—helps us to clarify our values, set our priorities, and plan wisely for the changes that aging brings.

This "live for today" attitude exemplifies a phenomenon that may surprise many—even though it's quite common: people aged sixty and older generally have a greater sense of well-being than younger people do. In fact, many surveys of happiness conducted in developed countries over the past few decades consistently show a "U-shaped" pattern. That is, the percentage of people on either end of the age spectrum report the highest levels of well-being, while folks in the middle fall to the lower levels.

In one large U.S. study by Brookings Institute scholars Carol Graham and Milena Nikolova, for example, self-reported measurement of happiness was high for eighteen- to twenty-one-year-olds and dropped steadily until about age forty.[2] Then the pattern began to reverse—gradually climbing back up, reaching its highest point at age ninety-eight. One infographic placed the data on a horizontal timeline with each end curving upward, appropriately, to form a smile.[3]

These findings seem to defy popular culture, which typically equates happiness with traits such as youthful energy, physical prowess, and earning power. They also appear to contradict research that shows increased depression among older people as they experience chronic illness, death of loved ones, and other losses common for the elderly. But aging also brings that broadened perspective Meredith describes—an attitude that naturally allows greater acceptance of ourselves and our lives—no matter how difficult circumstances may be at times. It's not that conditions necessarily get better as we age. It's that we have the chance to let go of our aspirations and be more realistic about life's ups and downs.

This idea that expecting less can lead to greater happiness in old age was actually proven by a young German economist at Princeton University a few years ago. Hannes Schwandt analyzed data from a long-term study of twenty-three thousand people who were surveyed from 1991 to 2004 regarding their current life satisfaction and their expectations for life five years into the future.[4] Because the data was collected over several years, he was able to learn about people's aspirations and then see how things turned out. He discovered that young adults had high aspirations that were often unmet, leading to lower life satisfaction. But older people had just the opposite experience. By age fifty, they had been disappointed so often that they abandoned hope that life would improve. In other words, they lowered their expectations to align with their experience. While this may sound sad, the study reveals a wonderful silver lining: life actually improved for many of the older folks over time. And when it did, they were more likely to be surprised and delighted with the result.

Now at the University of Zurich, Dr. Schwandt described the phenomenon in the *Harvard Business Review* : "People come to terms with how their life is playing out. . . . This combination of accepting life and feeling less regret about the past is what makes life satisfaction increase again. And since people over 50 tend to *underestimate* their future satisfaction, these increases come as an unexpected pleasant surprise, which further raises satisfaction levels."[5]

As we let go of expectations, we no longer have to figure out who we want to become or what else we want to accomplish. We let go of striving for advancement or status. We're not consumed with the obsessions of early adulthood and midlife—chasing after a multitude of goals in work, family, and recreational life. We choose activities based on what we *want* to do—not what we *have* to do to earn a living or meet other people's demands. It's not that older people don't have goals; they do. But often their aspirations are more focused and more achievable, resulting in a greater sense of happiness. Comfortable in our own skin, we can relax, finally zeroing in on activities aligned with our truest values.

It's also the time of life you can best appreciate this wisdom, sometimes attributed to author Elizabeth Gilbert:

> We spend our twenties and thirties so worried about what everyone
> is thinking about us. Then we get into our forties and fifties, and we
> finally start to be free, because we decide we don't give a damn what
> anyone thinks of us. But you will not be completely free until your
> sixties and seventies, when you will finally realize this liberating
> truth: nobody was ever thinking about you anyhow. [6]

Meanwhile, calamities common to youth become less likely. Having
learned our lessons, we sidestep the kind of trouble that may have
caused terrible stress in younger years. Old people are not immune to
financial risk, infidelity, overwork, overconsumption, and a host of other
risky behaviors. But many of us recognize our mistakes and can avoid
repeating the worst ones.

We're also finding more meaning in simpler but deeper gratifica-
tions—activities like caring for grandchildren, spending time in nature,
nurturing a pet, helping others, especially friends and neighbors, or just
sharing laughs and a good meal with relatives. Young people may see
their grandparents' lives as a boring, contracted existence. But Stanford
University Psychology Professor Laura Carstensen believes that older
people tend to place a high priority on relationships and activities that
bring near-term feelings of well-being for good reason: they know that
life is short and getting shorter. "As people age and increasingly per-
ceive time as finite, they attach less importance to goals that expand
their horizons and greater importance to goals from which they derive
emotional meaning," Dr. Carstensen explained in the journal *Science*. [7]

We've also learned that disappointment, disability, and loss are part
of life. So when they happen, they are less shocking. We can do a lot to
stave off illness, but we know that if we live long enough, we'll experience life-threatening diseases and functional decline. We know we're
going to lose some of the people we love most. When that happens, we
grieve and learn to accept grieving as natural and normal, as part of
being human. We're also beginning to realize and accept the inevitabil-
ity of our own death and dying.

To live fully despite such threats and losses, we must give up the
argument that we and our loved ones will be the exceptions. Nobody
gets out of here alive. And what may sound like gallows humor to the

young rings true for elders: the happiest older people seem to understand that life is limited.

At age eighty-seven, Erik Erikson—the midcentury psychoanalyst famous for observing the stages of psychosocial development—described the prime developmental task of old age to the *New York Times* this way: "You've got to learn to accept the law of life, and face the fact that we disintegrate slowly." To avoid despair, we must also develop "ego-integrity," he explained. That is, we must be able to look back and know that our lives have been "complete."[8]

Perhaps that's why so many older people find satisfaction in focusing on the needs of others—especially the next generation. They want to do good work, leaving the world better for future generations.

GIVING TO THE FUTURE

That's how it was for my longtime friend and father-in-law "Grandpa" Bob Zufall, a urologist who started a free clinic for disadvantaged people in Dover, New Jersey, near the same town where he had practiced for decades. He and his wife, Kay, hatched the idea after two tours of duty in Peru with CARE, the international relief organization. While Bob shared his skills with a Peruvian surgeon, Kay taught English at the local hospital. They enjoyed the experience immensely and considered returning to Peru after Bob retired from his successful medical practice in 1990.

But once that day came, the couple realized how much help was needed in their own community. At that time—as today—more than half of Dover's population was of Mexican, Colombian, Dominican, or Puerto Rican descent, and many of their neighbors lacked adequate health care. So Bob and Kay arranged to set up a one-room clinic in the offices of a nonprofit organization serving their town's Latino population. Bob would provide the care, and Kay would handle the business end.

Bob is now ninety-one years old. I asked him recently why he didn't just buy golf clubs and retire to the country club like so many happily retired professionals do. "Fortunately, I'm a lousy golfer," he laughed.[9]

He also said he believes that retirement is a perfect time to ask yourself this question: "What needs to be done that you *can* do and that you *enjoy* doing?"

Bob recognizes health professionals may have an easier time than others finding satisfying volunteer work. After all, affordable, high-quality health care is in short supply nearly worldwide. But, as Bob reminded me, the world also needs dedicated language teachers, carpenters, computer programmers, gardeners, and so on. That's why millions of older people everywhere are finding ways to "pay it forward." Whether they're caring for children in their own families, volunteering for mission-driven nonprofit organizations, or simply practicing "random acts of kindness," they find meaning through connecting to a world larger than themselves.

The Zufalls found their satisfaction was that tiny one-room clinic. "We hung up a curtain and rolled in a single exam table," Bob remembers fondly.

At first, the Dover Free Clinic was open just one night a week. The couple paid for basic medications out of their own pocket. Word spread quickly, however, so Bob and Kay soon extended their hours and started charging five dollars per visit to cover the cost of basic supplies. They also changed the name to the Dover Community Clinic and recruited a few more volunteers, including some of Bob's retired physician friends. Many were weary of the red tape involved in running their own medical practices, but they still loved seeing patients. This clinic gave them the opportunity to avoid the administrative burden while pursuing their passion: providing primary care for people who really needed and appreciated their services.

The clinic also gave the volunteers an opportunity to expand their horizons. Having spent his entire career in urology, Bob was now learning about primary care generally, and pediatrics in particular. His lessons came from textbooks, medical education classes, and consultation with the other physicians.

"I remember somebody asking one of the volunteers, 'What do you think of Dr. Zufall as a pediatrician?' And this guy said, 'He's like a really good third- or fourth-year resident.' I was kind of proud of that," Bob laughs.

The clinic also attracted the attention of the state board of health. "I was a little embarrassed," says Bob, recalling the health commissioner's tour of their humble operation. "But the commissioner looked around the room and said, 'I like it!' And he gave us $100,000."

With this first grant in hand, the clinic moved to a larger facility in a nearby church basement and hired its first paid staff. They also received a small "start-up" grant from the Robert Wood Johnson Foundation, the highly regarded New Jersey–based national health foundation with a special interest in improving local community health and services. Over the next twenty years, the clinic continued to grow and fulfill its mission of providing basic care for Dover's underserved populations. Eventually, it became a Federally Qualified Health Center, attracting enough federal and philanthropic support to open six separate sites in North and Central New Jersey. By 2011, the community board decided to rename the enterprise Zufall Health Centers, honoring Bob and Kay for their vision and long-term commitment.

Bob continued this medical practice for eighteen years after the organization was founded, and in 2015 he was still serving on its board. Kay served until she became disabled with Alzheimer's disease. She died in 2014 at age eighty-seven.

I recently asked Bob to compare his two careers—the one in private-practice urology before retirement, and the one as a volunteer primary care physician in a public health clinic after he retired.

"It was like apples and oranges," he tells me. "I had a nice career as a urologist and I was satisfied. I did good operations and I helped people. But with the Dover Health Center, I helped *a lot more* people."

Thinking of Erik Erikson's ideal of feeling "complete," I dig deeper, asking Bob if his service to others has affected the way he thinks about himself at this period of his life—that is, in old-old age, the time when people are anticipating death. The question does not surprise him. In fact, he assured me he's been thinking about his own death quite a lot lately.

"When you're a young person, you think, 'I am going to live forever—just like I am, thirty years old, vigorous, athletic, and sexy.' And then you get to be my age and you understand that aging is gradual dying."

The thought reminds him of this line from poet Wallace Stevens: "Death is the mother of beauty."

"He's telling us that things are beautiful to the extent we can understand they are limited," Bob explains, and I can see that my old friends

Bob and Meredith—though separated by twenty years—are on the same track. Both understand that life gets better when you accept that your time may be short.

And what does Bob's service to the community clinic add to the mix?

"It *does* make me feel better about dying to know that I have done something good with my life," he says.

Then, with total humility, he adds, "We all have feelings about things that we may have done wrong or stupidly. But as long as we're alive, we can still do good things—the things we may not have had time for earlier."

He's also pleased that his contribution will live on after he's gone. "One of my happiest thoughts is that the health center will continue in Dover," he says. "And maybe it could inspire others to serve the same way too."

For me, Bob's story provides an extraordinary example of Erik Erikson's concept of generativity—that is, giving away your time, talent, and resources to benefit future generations. The results are good not only for communities. Benefits accrue to those who give of themselves.[10] Through volunteerism, we keep and build our skills, learn new things, and meet new people. We also avoid the loneliness, regret, and boredom that can happen in later years.

This is the experience of "ego-integrity" that Erikson wrote about—the satisfaction of having made our lives compete.

WHAT IS "NORMAL AGING"?

In learning to accept the changes that come with age, many people wonder, "What's normal?" I remember my friend and patient Marcus Aquino, the former university administrator, arriving at my office after his retirement and announcing, "Aging is not for sissies!"

He was talking about his own elderly mother, who had just moved in with him, bringing with her a host of health concerns. But I knew he was also concerned about himself. He was experiencing a minor heart irregularity, and he had absolutely no interest in slowing down. He intended to keep golfing, sailing, playing music, and volunteering in the community. He would begin his retirement fully engaged, maintaining his characteristic strength and vitality. There would be no complaining, no "sissy-dom" about it. He simply wanted information about what was normal and what was not.

Most of us know, for example, that hearing, vision, and memory typically grow weaker over time. We can expect to have a harder time remembering some people's names; this is a common part of aging and not usually a sign of a degenerative brain disease. We also know that our joints tend to wear down, so knee and back pain becomes more common. But how do we know when the changes we're experiencing are just a usual part of aging to be tolerated—and not a disease or medical condition that requires intervention? Is it normal to become slower getting up the stairs? To have a hard time remembering your own grandchildren's names? To lose muscle mass? To have trouble sleeping through the night?

There are no "one-size-fits-all" answers to such questions. But it can help to view old age the same way we think about another big transition in life—adolescence. This occurred to me as I passed a middle school recently and saw a group of twelve- to fifteen-year-olds waiting for the bus. There was huge variation in the teenagers' shapes and sizes. Some looked like young adults, but others were still just little kids, showing no signs of sexual maturity. Although very different, they were all "normal" for their age. By the time they graduate from high school, the outliers will catch up. But at this period in their lives, the group showed lots of differences.

That's the way it is for older people too. From about age twenty to sixty, there's not as much variation in the way our bodies and minds function. With the exception of women in menopause, adults in the middle years are not undergoing a lot of intense, age-related changes. But once we reach sixty, the range of normal begins to increase. This is true for factors easy to track and spot—things like wrinkling and hair, vision, and memory loss. It's also true for measures that are not so noticeable—things like kidney function, bone density, height, or walking speed. And depending on what's being measured, abnormalities are usually only a problem if you're on the very high or very low end of an extremely wide normal range.

I believe it's important for everybody—lay people, health care providers, caregivers, and so on—to expect a wide range of normal in aging. Accepting this can help us avoid "medicalizing" normal changes of aging—that is, misinterpreting such changes as diseases that require medical attention. Examples include decreased levels of estrogen in women following menopause or lower levels of testosterone in men. Perceiving these and other age-related conditions as problems that need to be "cured" can lead to unwarranted and sometimes harmful overtreatment. In their 2005 book *Selling Sickness: How the World's Biggest Pharmaceutical Companies Are Turning Us All into Patients*, journalist Ray Moynihan and health policy researcher Alan Cassels described such forms of medicalization as "disease mongering—extending the boundaries of illness to expand markets for new products."[11] Such marketing manipulates our culture's fears of aging and obsession with staying forever young. People who fall prey not only waste money on ineffective measures; they may also suffer from unnecessary medical treatments that have risky side effects. But you can avoid such exploitation by learning all you can about normal aging processes. Seek information from independent, objective sources rather than corporations with drugs and products to sell. And understand that some changes are simply to be expected and accepted over time.

Does this mean you should ignore symptoms you find troublesome? Not at all.

It makes sense to talk with your health care team about changes that worry you. Doing so allows them to help you manage minor issues while ruling out medical problems that really can benefit from treatment. Your providers may also give you tips for staying well. But don't be afraid to ask lots of questions, and push back if you feel you're getting too much medicine or too much intervention for changes that seem to be just a normal part of life as we age.

LIMIT STRESS, INCLUDING TOO MUCH CARE

It's also important to understand how stress can be harmful to well-being as we age. Minimizing stress is especially crucial as people grow very old and naturally lose their bodies' inherent tendency toward homeostasis—that is, its capacity to coordinate internal systems such as pulse, blood pressure, body temperature, and so on, keeping them within a healthy range. For younger people, environmental factors such as extremely hot weather or a heart-thumping emotional upset don't generally pose a danger because younger bodies can more easily adjust.

But the older we get, the harder it is to maintain internal stability. As a result, big, stressful changes are more likely to interfere with physical and mental health. That source of stress can be physical or emotional.

Understanding older people's slower adaptation to change is especially significant when addressing very elderly patients' symptoms, adjusting their medications, or helping them decide where to live. As a physician who understands aging, homeostasis, and the need to avoid sudden, stressful changes, I have learned to use the "slow care" approach that Dennis McCullough describes in his 2008 book *My Mother, Your Mother: Embracing "Slow Medicine," the Compassionate Approach to Caring for Your Aging Loved Ones.*[12]

I try not to recommend too many adjustments too quickly, avoiding extreme changes except in dire circumstances. I also want to help my elderly patients stay out of hospitals whenever possible; our research has shown that an inpatient stay—with all its unfamiliarity and disruptions in daily routine—is a source of great stress and can increase an elderly person's risk for dementia. It can also put them at risk for overtreatment.

As Dr. McCullough wrote for *Dartmouth Medicine*, American medicine too often subjects elderly patients to "death by intensive care." Patients are

> subjected to enduring impersonal medical protocols in strange, disorienting surroundings or stranded in limbo on life-support machines while their families hover in waiting rooms, uncertain how to help. . . . This high drama happens for some, but much more commonly elders suffer the accumulating burdens of illness and exhausting medical regimens that extract all their available energy and time, leaving nothing left for living beyond a "medicalized" life.[13]

I am reminded of a series of unfortunate events that befell my own patient Roger Brooks when he was in his early nineties. Roger was married to a nurse and former colleague of mine, Charlotte Brooks—also my patient. I got a call one evening from a local hospital that he was in the emergency department with chest pain. The ER doctor wanted to call in a cardiologist.

"Are you sure?" I asked, before stating the obvious: "Mr. Brooks is a very old man. It's highly unlikely that this pain is due to an emergent heart condition. What are we going to gain?"

As his primary care physician, I also knew Roger would not be interested in extraordinary measures such as heart surgery to extend his life at this age. So what was the point of doing an invasive, expensive diagnostic procedure? Although chest pain was unusual for Roger, it's common for men in their nineties to have such symptoms with no attributable cause.

The emergency physician understood this but also needed to do his best to respond to Roger and Charlotte, who were in his exam room and looking for answers. So despite some reluctance from me, Roger, and Charlotte, we eventually all agreed to call the cardiologist, who promptly ordered a cardiac catheterization, a procedure that involves inserting a long, thin tube into an artery or vein in the groin and threading it through blood vessels to the heart, where images can show how well the heart is working. As was routine, a nurse was also called in to provide a Foley catheter, a tube that's inserted into the penis to keep the bladder drained during the procedure. But Roger, like many men his age, had an enlarged prostate gland, which made the Foley very difficult to insert. After several attempts and the involvement of a urologist, the catheter was finally placed—but not before the process, which turned out to be complicated and painful, caused irreparable damage to Roger's urethra.

Eventually, the cardiac procedure was completed and the images were analyzed. Roger's tests showed no sign of heart disease. "He's got the coronary arteries of a thirty- or forty-year-old man," the cardiologist said. But along the way, the team found something totally unexpected: a suspicious small mass on Roger's pancreas. It was a classic "incidentaloma"—in Roger's case, the unexpected discovery of a cancer when doctors were not even looking. Roger's cancer had nothing to do with the chest pain that brought him to the hospital, but he went home with a terminal diagnosis anyway. He also went home with a catheter permanently inserted into his bladder and a bag he would wear to catch his urine for the rest of his life.

Understandably indignant, Roger told me afterward he would never set foot in a hospital again. And thanks to the home-based care he subsequently received, he was able to avoid inpatient and most clinic visits from that point on. But we always wondered how his last years might have played out had he not gone to the emergency department that night. What if he and Charlotte and all the care providers involved had been practicing "slow care"? Given that he was over ninety, what if all had taken more of a "wait and see" approach, recognizing that it can be "normal" for a very old man to feel chest pain and for the chest pain to then dissipate?

Roger actually lived for nearly three years after that event, far exceeding expectations for someone diagnosed with pancreatic cancer. But once he had a permanent urinary catheter, he no longer felt comfortable traveling or going out to dinner, to the opera, and to other activities that he and Charlotte so savored. To their credit, the couple lived those final years together with remarkable grace and pleasure. Roger loved old movies, and they had a tremendous library of books and music that they enjoyed. They focused on their relationship, close friends, and making their days at home together as rich as possible. To me, they were the epitome of wise elders who accept the limitations of illness and aging, learning to treasure each remaining day as it comes.

TAKING CHANGES IN STRIDE

Wherever you are on the spectrum of "normal aging," there is absolutely no reason to give up efforts to maintain your strength and vitality just because you recognize that certain functions naturally decline with age. Habits like daily exercise, eating a healthy diet, socializing, and doing activities that challenge your brain are all important for building "reserves" that will keep you going—a concept we'll explore in the chapters ahead.

And remember, you can almost always take steps to improve your sense of well-being. At the same time, it's good to know that change happens and to take these shifts in stride.

I'm reminded of my own experience mountaineering, a pastime I've enjoyed since I was a boy growing up in the shadow of Oregon's Mount Hood. In adulthood, I spent countless weekends with my climbing buddies, scaling peaks in Western Washington's North Cascades. But by the time my friends and I reached our sixties, many of us no longer had the strength and endurance for the kind of technical ascents we used to do. It would be a lie to say I don't miss it, because I do. In fact, I still daydream of being on some remote Cascade peak at sunset. Having just returned from an exhilarating ascent, my friends and I are enjoying a meal prepared over a camp stove. With our tents pitched on a permanent snowfield, our world is turning pink-orange with an evening alpine glow. But wait! I bring myself back to reality, remembering, "I don't do that anymore."

At age sixty-seven, I could have chosen to spend a lot of time reconditioning so that I might return to mountain climbing. I've seen others my age do this, focusing their time and energy on becoming superathletic. But that would take an immense effort that would upset the balance I'm aiming for and distract me from other important interests—my family, my friends, travel, gardening, further research, and writing. It would also expose me to more risk than I want at this time of life.

And so I look for a satisfying middle ground. I still exercise vigorously—just not as vigorously as I did when I was younger. By staying reasonably fit, I can still spend time in the Cascades taking invigorating hikes and skiing. It's not mountain climbing, but it's better than becoming so discouraged that I quit being active. I've seen this happen with former athletes who can't seem to dial back their activities (shorter bike rides, tamer ski runs, etc.). Sadly, they give up sports altogether and become sedentary, losing their ability to be active much earlier than they otherwise would.

I also think of my friend Meredith, who started walking half marathons in her early fifties. By her late sixties, she developed chronic pain in her big toe, a common spot for age-related osteoarthritis. Rather than quit, she saw a physical therapist who recommended an orthotic shoe insert and taught her how to tape her foot—both of which reduced her pain. She also learned to pace herself, walking fewer miles in the days leading up to a race so that her joints would be well rested.

"It's a little discouraging, but I figure you can't let these things stop you," Meredith says. "I don't want to be the person who says, 'I've got arthritis in my feet, so I can't do that.' To me, *that* would be the definition of an *old* person. I may get there, but I'm not there yet."

WHAT IS "SUCCESSFUL AGING"?

Although it's challenging to define normal aging, researchers are making great progress at finding out what improves older people's well-being. In 1987, for example, researchers John W. Rowe and Robert L. Kahn came up with a model of "successful aging" that includes three main components: (1) low probability of disease and disease-related disability; (2) high capacity for thinking and physical function; and (3) active engagement with life.[14]

While such models help us define and measure health in aging, they do not shed much light on issues that would help older people clarify their values, accept changes, and plan for the future. They don't tell us how people feel about longevity, independence, work, and family relationships, for example. For this reason, Rowe and Kahn's ideas, which seem so logical, have been criticized as promoting a denial of aging—as though we could continue to grow old without eventually experiencing disease and disability.

I'll never forget an older patient, a retired circus worker, whom I cared for in the late 1970s. He had diabetes and lots of problems, including a life-threatening infection that had damaged his kidneys. I knew he would eventually need kidney dialysis. But over several years, he repeatedly told me, "Doc, whatever happens, don't put me on that artificial kidney. I couldn't stand being tied up to a machine."

As he approached that dreaded transition, however—to my utter surprise—he changed his mind. He had made a new friend who gave him a new purpose in life—enough so that he decided to accept the dialysis. Sadly, he did not live long after that; a heart attack took his life just six months into dialysis. But from what I could see, those six months were happy ones he might have missed if he had not been willing to accept the limitations of his condition and its treatment. By resetting his priorities and perspective, he experienced a kind of "successful aging" that conventional assessments would have missed.

It was this kind of real-world experience that our research team from the University of Washington and Group Health Research Institute had in mind several years ago when we sought to better understand older people's ideas about what it meant to age "successfully." Led by UW's Elizabeth A. Phelan, the team surveyed about 1,200 people enrolled in our ACT study and 717 people in a similar group of Seattle-area Japanese American elders. The average age of those surveyed was eighty years old, and all were free from dementia.

Before we did our research, we expected to find differences in the two groups—presumably because Japanese culture reveres aging more than the typical culture in Seattle. We were surprised, however, to find that the results of the survey were exactly the same for both the ACT subjects and the Japanese American group.

We analyzed the survey results of both groups (see table 3.1), concluding that successful aging can be observed across multiple dimensions: physical, functional, social, psychological, and chronological.

You may be surprised to see that participants rated "living a very long time" as the least important value. On average, they felt it was more important to avoid dysfunction and pain from chronic illness. But even more than this, they wanted to keep learning, contributing, and being involved in other people's lives. They highly valued relationships with their friends and family. And most importantly, they wanted to stay in good health until close to death, living independently and not being a burden to their families.

These survey results may or may not align with your feelings about growing older. But you may find it helpful to look at the items in table 3.1 and think carefully about your own wishes and priorities. How important is it to you to live independently? To be close to friends and family? To continue contributing through work or volunteer activities? If you had to rank all these items, what would be at the top of your list, in the middle, or at the bottom? Is "living a long time" your most valued desire? Or would it be more important for you to be able to meet all of your own needs?

PLAN TO ENJOY THE RIDE

Answering such questions may give you a clearer sense of the changes ahead and how you'd like to prepare for them. Aging well is like planning for any important journey. If you can visualize the trip and predict what you'll need in order to be safe and comfortable, you're going to have a lot more joy along the way.

At the same time, it pays to stay flexible. In any journey—but especially a long one—the decisions you make at the beginning of the trip may not be the ones you'll want to cling to later on. So like any wise traveler, you may want to periodically reassess your wishes and priorities as time goes by.

Table 3.1.   Perceptions of Older Adults Regarding Successful Aging

	Percent of ACT participants who rated this item important to successful aging
Remaining in good health until close to death	94.9
Being able to take care of myself until close to the time of my death	94.7
Being able to cope with the challenges of my later years	92.8
Being able to meet all of my needs and some of my wants	91.6
Being able to act according to my own inner standards and values	91.6
Being able to make choices about things that affect how I age, like my diet, exercise, and smoking	91.5
Having friends and family who are there for me	90.2
Remaining free of chronic disease	90.1
Staying involved with the world and people around me	87.5
Feeling good about myself	85.1
Feeling satisfied with my life the majority of the time	84.2
Not feeling lonely or isolated	83.5
Adjusting to changes that are related to aging	83.4
Continuing to learn new things	78.6
Having a sense of peace when thinking about the fact that I will not live forever	72.0
Having the kind of genes (heredity) that help me age well	69.6
Feeling I have been able to influence others' lives in positive ways	67.2
Having no regrets about how I lived my life	66.9
Being able to work in paid or volunteer activities after usual retirement age (sixty-five)	50.2
Living a very long time	29.1

And finally, you'll want to be as physically strong, mentally stable, and optimistic as you can be. This will keep you resilient—able to bounce back from any difficulties you encounter. Ideally, you'll have the financial resources and assistance necessary to feel secure. And because you'll want to have fun—and not be lonely—it's best to have people around you to share the road.

In the chapters ahead we'll explore how to build and maintain such reserves so you can anticipate a very good ride.

4

BUILD YOUR RESERVES FOR RESILIENCE

In thousands of conversations over many decades, I've heard my patients and study participants express the same wish for old age: they want to live independently in good health, postponing serious illness and disability until the very end.

Scientists call this "compression of morbidity"—a term Stanford University's James Fries first used in 1980 to suggest that most diseases of old age could be squeezed into a short period at the end of life.[1] He revisited the idea in 2011, showing that subsequent research proved this to be a good approach for healthy aging.[2]

In Japan, the concept is called "pin pin korori"—a phrase that combines words for a healthy and energetic life ("pin pin") with a word for dying quickly and painlessly ("korori"). Elderly Japanese visit temples or shrines to pray for "PPK"—healthy longevity followed by a good death.

The idea is popular for good reason: it gives you as much time as possible to pursue your proverbial bucket list. Whether you spend that time building a free clinic like Dr. Bob Zufall did or ballroom dancing like Evangeline Shuler, it's up to you. You get to choose your own adventure, unencumbered by sickness and disability. With less time spent dependent on others, you avoid the worry that was commonly expressed in our survey on successful aging: "being a burden" to others.

And here's the good news for boomers. Science suggests our generation now has a better chance than previous ones to experience old age with less illness and disability. This is due in large part to socioeconomic and medical advances that allow us to prevent or postpone common conditions, especially cardiovascular disease and maybe even Alzheimer's.

But this opportunity is by no means universal or guaranteed. Our longevity and wellness still depend on many individual factors, such as our inherited risks and our lifestyle. So while more and more boomers can now *see* the brass ring—that is, a longer, healthier old age—only some of us will get the chance to grab that prize. I believe the advantage will go to those who can anticipate the mental, physical, and social reserves they'll need for old age. And in the next four chapters, we'll be exploring how to go about building those reserves.

LEARNING FROM ONE PARENT'S EXPERIENCE

Paul Leland, fifty-six, is an architect and avid bicyclist who was just diagnosed with high cholesterol—a trait that he may have inherited from his father, Tom, who died at age eighty-nine. Paul never expected his dad to live that long because Tom had so many chronic health problems made worse by his obesity.

"For years, I would travel back to the Midwest to visit my folks, and each time I said good-bye to my dad, I thought it might be the last time I would see him," Paul said. [3]

An ex-smoker with type 2 diabetes, Tom suffered his first heart attack at age fifty-one when Paul was a teenager. Even after bypass surgery, Tom's heart problems continued. He also had chronic digestive problems and painful arthritis in his knees.

A father of five, Tom had been a police officer when he was younger, but he spent most of his adult life in sedentary, high-pressure sales jobs. Once his health problems started, he was often on disability, which made it tough for this family to pay their bills. The stress seemed to fuel Tom's physical problems, and his illnesses worsened his stress.

"My dad just seemed to go from one health crisis to another," Paul remembered. There were more heart attacks and many hospitalizations and procedures involving his heart and his colon.

Paul believes his dad probably suffered from undiagnosed depression, which is common for people with heart disease and diabetes. Overmedication might have been a problem as well. But Paul could never convince his dad to seek counseling. "For guys his age, there was a lot of stigma about seeing a shrink," said Paul.

Instead, his dad retreated to his bedroom, watching television twelve hours a day or more.

"When I was little, he would spend weekends working on old cars or taking us fishing, but as his health got worse, he let that go by the wayside," Paul said.

With little exercise but a lot of snacking, Tom put on more weight, which made all of his health problems worse. The heavier he got, the harder it was for him to walk on painfully swollen, arthritic knees. And the more pain he had, the less he wanted to move.

By his midseventies, Tom started having intermittent problems with his memory—issues his doctor attributed to transient ischemic attacks (TIAs) or mini-strokes. By his eighties, he had mild dementia, probably the result of ongoing cardiovascular problems.

Tom lived his last six years in an assisted living facility with his wife. Because of his mobility problems and dementia, he rarely wanted to leave their apartment. He died in a hospital after complications from surgery for a bowel obstruction.

Over the years, I have known many patients with health histories similar to Tom's. They live a surprisingly long life thanks to modern medical care, but their quality of life is not good. Dr. Fries warned about cases like this in his landmark paper decades ago: advanced life expectancy allows patients to live longer, but they're being saddled with years of disability and dependency. As some seniors would say, they're "adding years to their lives but not life to their years." It's exactly the opposite outcome seniors in our successful aging survey said they wanted for themselves.

That's not to say that all was misery for Tom. "My dad was happy at times—especially when the grandkids came around," said Paul. "But I think he spent most of his time struggling with his pain and discomfort or trying to escape it."

If Tom had had any goals for his later years, he didn't share them with his son. "He used to talk about buying a used motorhome and fixing it up—maybe taking it on a cross-country trip," Paul recalled. But with his health problems and financial pressures, that dream never materialized.

As for his own aspirations, Paul is adamant he won't follow his dad's example. "I have stuff to do—I want to travel especially," he said. Retirement is still a few years away, but Paul and his wife hope to do some cycling tours in Australia and Europe. They want to stay as active as possible as long as they can. "We don't want to spend our last thirty years too sick to do anything but watch TV."

LET'S DO THIS DIFFERENTLY

With his presumed inherited risk for cardiovascular disease, Paul knows that he needs to take his health seriously. Fortunately, like many boomers, Paul has several advantages that many in his father's generation never enjoyed.

For one, Paul's education gives him a basic understanding of the science behind today's health advice. He realizes a healthy lifestyle can help him counter his inherited risk. That's why he never smoked, and why he takes an "activist" stance by exercising regularly, eating right, and taking the drugs his doctor prescribed for his cholesterol. Contrast this with Tom and his cohort. Like so many men of his generation, Tom started smoking when the navy provided sailors with cigarettes, standard practice for servicemen during World War II. He was forty years old and addicted to tobacco before the U.S. surgeon general started stamping warning labels on cigarette packs in 1965. Also back then, there was little understanding of the way nutrition and physical activity affects health. To many in Tom's generation, daily workouts were only for "health nuts" like sixties television exercise guru Jack LaLanne.

Paul also has the advantage of knowing he could actually live quite long—maybe into his nineties. That awareness may be an incentive for investing in prevention—being physically active, eating better, managing his stress. Tom, on the other hand, probably imagined a much closer death—especially after he had his first heart attack in the early 1970s, when mortality rates for cardiovascular disease were much higher. "Nobody imagined that my dad would live to be eighty-nine," said Paul.

And finally, to paraphrase the Rolling Stones, time is on Paul's side. As you'll learn in the chapters ahead, the process of building reserves for old age begins before birth and continues through childhood, adolescence, and the adult years. Born to middle-class Americans in the prosperous 1950s, Paul has health advantages over his dad, who was raised during the Great Depression. And even in middle age, Paul still has plenty of time to amass reserves for use later on.

IT'S LIKE A MARATHON

To live comfortably and independently, as so many seniors wish to do, requires preservation of four basic functions—thinking clearly, moving safely, hearing, and seeing. Over time, the body's aging processes chip away at these abilities. But as an activist ager, you can adapt to such changes, building reserves to maintain function, staving off disability as long as possible. Your reserves may include many factors, such as your brain cells, your intellect, your blood vessels, your friendships, your muscles, your savings account—*all* of it.

It may help to think of yourself as an athlete getting ready for a marathon. Instead of a morning race, however, you're preparing for decades of senior living. If you want to make it to the finish line, you need resources to last the entire race.

The more reserves you have going into old age, the more resilient you'll be when facing late-life challenges. By resilience, I mean the ability to withstand physical or emotional setbacks, to recover from them, and to keep going. Like a tree that has weathered many storms, resilient people have the ability to "bend, not break" under pressure. They can bounce back from adversity, sometimes stronger than ever before.

Growing old presents plenty of opportunities to put your resilience to the test. As my patient Marcus Aquino said, "Aging is not for sissies." Trials range from serious illness, to the diminishment of skills and senses, to the loss of many dear friends and relatives. But if you come to aging fully resourced, activated, and aware of the challenges ahead, you're going to have a much richer, more satisfying experience.

Many of my patients have possessed these qualities. But I can think of one whose stalwart comeback in old age was particularly remarkable. He was Ben Stevenson, a professor of education who became my patient after retiring to Washington State in 1972 to be near his daughter.

Ben was born in 1906 on a farm in Kansas, where he rode his horse to school each day and enjoyed playing sports and reciting poetry. He became a high school teacher and coach before earning his doctorate in 1932 and establishing a career in public school law and finance. While waiting for jobs during the Great Depression, he and his brother broke and sold wild horses to earn money.

Through adulthood, Ben's life continued to be a rich mix of intellectual and physical challenges. In addition to his academic role, he traveled the world, serving as an education consultant to foreign governments. During summer vacations, he would return to the family farm to help his brother harvest hay. On a daily basis, he stayed vigorous by walking to work and gardening.

In retirement, he bought a small farm where he raised Arabian horses. He kept his mind engaged with reading, writing, and publishing poetry. He revised his textbook on school law.

As Ben grew older, the horses "kept him going," his son-in-law told me.[4] At age eighty-five, Ben's wife of fifty-six years passed away. But still, he kept caring for the horses.

Eventually, he found his large garden too demanding. But the horses were different. They gave him a way to connect with others—especially as he helped his grandchildren and others learn to ride. "He would tell them about things he used to do as a kid—little anecdotes," his son-in-law said. "It unified his life."

But one day, when Ben was ninety and tending to one of the horses, something went wrong with the lunge line. Somehow, Ben got caught in the rope and was knocked to the ground, suffering many nasty, ugly bruises and several broken ribs. He tried to care for himself at home with pain medication, but soon his bladder stopped working, so he went to the hospital, where he was admitted.

When I first saw him there, battered and confused, I was afraid he would not recover from the trauma of the accident, let alone return to his small farm. Most people his age, with injuries so severe, would not survive. But what happened over the next two months was nothing short of miraculous. Ben began to heal and regain his strength. After a few days, he was moved to the hospital rehabilitation floor, and then to an outpatient rehabilitation facility where he lived for a little over a month. Not only did he reclaim his bearings and mobility there; he also made many new friends among the patients and staff. After he was released, his new friends visited the farm to meet his beloved beasts.

Once home, Ben gradually increased his activity. Eventually he developed a routine of walking two to three miles a day. And for several more years, he was able to enjoy his horses—albeit with a lot of caution to prevent another accident. He had learned to accommodate his age while not abandoning one of his life's greatest joys.

Looking back, I think of all the "reserves" Ben had accumulated that allowed him to live independently for so long and then to recover from his terrible accident. I believe Ben started gathering reserves for his resilience in early childhood. He was a wiry guy of average build, but according to family lore he could do the work of a full-grown man when he was only twelve years old. He became a sought-after farmhand and high school athlete who stayed physically fit into adulthood. Little did he know how much that foundation of bone and muscle mass would come in handy when he was ninety and older, and while healing from his injuries.

But Ben's strength would not have mattered if he had not had enough brain reserve to stay mentally well and independent in his nineties. More than half of all people suffer dementia by age ninety-five, but not Ben. His brain was in good working order, perhaps because he had kept his mind active so much of his life—not only during his career teaching, but also into retirement, when he was consulting, writing, and publishing poetry. Like many resilient seniors who recover from the stress of illness or dangerous medications that cause confusion, he was able to "bend but not break." His social reserves were also a benefit. Without the support of his kids, grandkids, and neighbors, he might not have been able to go back home.

Once Ben did return, he was able to live independently again for almost another year. After that, he went to Oregon for a few years to live with his sister until she became too frail to live at home. Then Ben moved back to Washington to an assisted living facility.

I had the pleasure of attending Ben's one hundredth birthday party, where he entertained the crowd with a witty poem about his life, "past, present, and future." He lived another year after that and died comfortably at 101.

In the next three chapters, you'll learn about ways to build, protect, and enhance your reserves for a resilient old age. Although I have divided these reserves into three categories—mental, physical, and social—and given each its own chapter, please keep in mind that these areas are all interrelated. Your strengths in one area surely contribute to your strengths in others. In fact, your well-being depends on your ability to build strengths across the board—a truth I didn't fully appreciate until quite late in my career. Now, thanks to the lessons I've learned working with patients like Ben Stevenson and many, many others, I understand how amazing the possibilities are. I can see the potential for postponing disability and enhancing quality of life even as you reach very old age.

5

BUILDING YOUR MENTAL RESERVES
Strengthening the Mind/Whole-Body Connection

It's Christmas Eve and Alice Howland is in her kitchen, skillfully preparing a multicourse family dinner. Played by Julianne Moore in the 2014 film *Still Alice*, she checks the turkey, chops butternut squash, and turns to her grown children just arriving from the airport. Graciously, she introduces herself to her son's new girlfriend.

"Hi, I'm Alice. I'm so happy you could join us. I really am."

Minutes later, her family gathers in the dining room. Alice enters, sets a large terrine on the table and—once again—introduces herself to her son's new girlfriend.

"Hi, I'm Alice. I'm so happy to meet you. It's wonderful you could join us."

The faux pas is subtly played, but it likely strikes a painful chord for audience members who recognize dementia. Like the girlfriend, we see something amiss and brace ourselves for many difficult scenes ahead.

Whether it's caused by the rare early-onset Alzheimer's disease depicted in *Still Alice* or a more common form of brain disease, most of our families are likely to be touched by dementia. Defined as "cognitive impairment sufficient enough to affect everyday functions," dementia currently happens to:

- one-third of people age eighty-five to ninety,
- one-half of those age ninety to ninety-five,

- and up to three-quarters of people age ninety-five and older.

With today's high prevalence of dementia, many baby boomers enter their elderly years "enlightened" by their experiences with their parents' generation. Boomers are, after all, the first generation to see so many in their parents' generation live beyond age eighty—and therefore to have more susceptibility to Alzheimer's disease and related chronic conditions.

Revelations in 1994 that former President Ronald Reagan had Alzheimer's disease brought the condition into the limelight. Public awareness has grown steadily since that time and will continue to grow in the years ahead. By studying the experience of today's elderly, researchers are amassing a growing body of scientific evidence about how these brain diseases can be prevented or at least postponed. We're also learning how to best care for loved ones living with these conditions.

If you're among the families affected, you may well remember that first moment you noticed something was seriously wrong with your parent, spouse, or relative. It wasn't a mere case of misplaced keys or forgetting the name of an old acquaintance. That kind of absentmindedness is normal and happens to everybody, especially as we age. More likely, the incident was alarming: Mom got lost coming home from the neighborhood grocery store—a short route she's traveled for years. Granddad couldn't play simple card games anymore because the deck just didn't make sense. Uncle George asked you the same question five times in ten minutes, and each time he acted like he had never raised the issue before.

Concern over such events is understandable. In fact, when physicians were asked in a survey which illness they feared most for themselves, their most common response was not what you might expect— say, cancer or a progressively crippling condition like Lou Gehrig's disease. Instead, it was Alzheimer's disease. The doctors had seen how dementia gradually takes away a person's ability to reason, to remember, and to communicate effectively, how it leads to personality changes, isolation, and eventually a sense that you've lost yourself. And they had seen people continue to live in this state for many years.

In addition, many people have an unfounded sense of resignation about dementia, believing that "senility" is a natural and unavoidable consequence of aging. Or they may mistakenly believe that all forms of dementia are inherited. They assume that if their parent had Alzheimer's disease, for example, they're doomed; there's nothing they or anyone can do to avoid the same fate.

CAUSE FOR OPTIMISM

Fortunately, for the vast majority of people, this kind of fatalism is uncalled for. As I'll explain in the pages ahead, current scientific evidence gives us hope that dementia can be prevented for many people— or at the very least, its onset can be delayed. In practical terms, this can mean that more people who get dementia begin experiencing it in very old age just a year or two before they die—maybe as a consequence of a brain disease like Alzheimer's or maybe from other age-related causes.

The key to long, dementia-free living is not a single "magic bullet" solution. There's no miracle drug or nutritional supplement you can take to prevent memory loss, no single set of games or online puzzles you can pursue to stave off dementia. Yes, we may wish for a simple cure, and that desire sustains a market for everything from parsley smoothies ("high vitamin content!") to the "scientifically proven" antiaging potions trumpeted in half-page newspaper ads and on the Internet. But that's not where the true, painstaking study of the aging mind has delivered us. Instead, we are finding answers through research into the lifelong experiences of large populations of real people who do and do not suffer from dementia. We are discovering that a combination of socioeconomic influences and healthy habits, taken together, can help us to build, preserve, and protect the brain's structure and ability to function well over time. Together, these factors create a reserve of brainpower, the magnitude of which determines how sharp our minds will be as we grow older.

The process of building so-called cognitive reserve starts in the womb as the architecture of a fetus's brain takes shape. It continues throughout childhood, adolescence, and adulthood as the structure of our brain modifies itself in response to our experiences and environment. Some experts believe such brain development can persist up until the time we die.

It may help to imagine the brain as a reservoir, gathering rainfall for later use over time. Many things happen throughout life to drain and refill your reservoir. In the same way, your body can build and maintain a reserve of brain cells and connective structures—allowing it to continually adapt and function, staying resilient in the face of stress and strain. The level of your reserve is likely to fall as the size of your brain inevitably shrinks with age. The brain naturally loses connections over time and its tissue degenerates, a process that can be observed on CT and MRI brain scans. But certain influences and activities may act like rain, replenishing your reserves for improved function—even in old age.

DISCOVERING THE PLASTIC BRAIN

The idea that the brain can keep developing as we age was not well established when I first began my research career in the 1970s. In fact, our knowledge of cognitive function, dementia, and ways to prevent degenerative diseases of the brain has expanded tremendously over the last four to five decades. This progress has been due in large part to amazing diagnostic tools and intense scientific interest in brain development, aging, and age-related brain diseases like Alzheimer's.

New imaging technologies have given us a window into the skull. To see inside the brain prior to the mid-1970s, scientists needed tissue samples obtained through autopsies, brain biopsies, or other invasive techniques. But development of computed tomography (i.e., CT scans) changed all that. Now we have amazingly powerful, noninvasive ways to collect detailed images of the brain, its interior structures, and diseases. Scientists are making discoveries based on analyzing millions of computerized images taken daily worldwide.

At the same time, researchers have been tracking large populations of aging adults, gathering tremendous knowledge by analyzing their family trees, medical records, and behaviors. We've gained a rich understanding of how brain health correlates with issues such as heredity, exercise, social activity, diet, and the use of drugs and alcohol.

When I started medical school in 1969, however, the profession had very little understanding of brain diseases and how to prevent them. In fact, the words *Alzheimer's disease* were hardly mentioned. The majority of people who were having problems with memory and cognitive function were elderly and simply labeled "senile"—a condition considered to be a normal manifestation of aging. We occasionally saw the rare patients in their fifties or sixties who were diagnosed with what we called "pre-senile dementia."

Neuroscientists of that era believed that brain growth pretty much stopped around late adolescence—about the same time that the hippocampus becomes fully developed. This small, seahorse-shaped structure in the brain is the key to memory, spatial orientation, and complex thinking and decision making. The common wisdom was that people reached a pinnacle of brain development in their late teens and then faced a slow, downhill slide. Once the hippocampus and other parts of the brain were completely formed, that was it; all we could do was try our best to maintain the brain's capacity. And what if someone lost brain cells due to a head injury, stroke, substance abuse, or other problems? That was very bad news because doctors believed little could be done to restore memory and other brain functions.

But since the 1970s, a remarkable body of work from researchers around the world has given us a new understanding. Their results show that the brain is actually quite malleable and always changing—a concept known as brain plasticity. In fact, we now know the brain can grow new cells and form new connections. Much like our muscles and other body parts, it can literally rebuild itself through repeated use and exercise, and it can repair itself following injury. This is welcome news for those studying brain health in the elderly—and for anybody who intends to grow old themselves. It means we can prevent or lessen problems like memory loss and dementia by focusing on mental, physical, and social activities that promote healthy brain development.

In my estimation, one of the most exciting discoveries about brain health appeared in 2011, showing *how* physical activity changes the brain. In this study led by Arthur Kramer, researchers from the University of Illinois and the University of Pittsburgh randomly assigned 120 people aged fifty-five to eighty to two groups. One group was instructed to walk vigorously around a track for forty minutes three times a week. (Keep in mind this was aerobic activity—i.e., so brisk that if you walked any faster you'd be out of breath.) The other performed a regular stretching routine. The scientists evaluated a variety of factors, including cognitive ability. They also did MRI brain scans and other lab tests, measuring a blood factor believed to stimulate brain-cell growth. After a year, the researchers found measurable improvement in the walking group's cognitive abilities.[1]

But here's the amazing part: For those assigned to the program of regular, aerobic walking exercises, high-end MRI brain scans showed growth in the average size of the hippocampus. Tests also showed an increase in the amount of a brain-stimulating growth factor in the walkers' blood. Published in the *Proceedings of the National Academy of Sciences*, this study not only demonstrated the benefit of physical activity; it also provided a potential explanation for how that benefit occurred: *aerobic exercise likely transformed the structure of the brain itself.*

LEARNING ABOUT THE GENETIC FOUNDATIONS OF ALZHEIMER'S DISEASE

One form of Alzheimer's disease—early-onset Alzheimer's—tends to run in families. This form of Alzheimer's appears before age sixty-five and is quite rare. Important research involving these families has provided knowledge and clues about its causes and has led to genetic tests for the condition. Further genetic research is underway and may help us target prevention and treatment for those at risk for this rare form of the disease.

In addition, there's hope that genetic research may someday help the far greater population of people at risk for the more common form of the disease—that which strikes people seventy-five and older. But far more research is needed before we can effectively screen or treat this much larger population of people.

Early research into the genetics of Alzheimer's disease began at the University of Washington and other institutions in the 1990s with scientists studying a group of American descendants of "the Volga Deutsch"—German immigrants who had settled in Russia's Volga Valley. These families had an unusually high proportion of people who developed early-onset Alzheimer's. By analyzing the DNA of about two hundred people in this group, the researchers discovered mutations in a gene referred to as the "presenilin" gene. Subsequent research in other populations found three gene abnormalities known as presenilin 1, presenilin 2, and the amyloid precursor protein gene—all of which are linked to the formation of harmful proteins in the brain.

Discoveries like these initially fostered great hope that we could soon find that elusive magic bullet for diagnosing and ultimately curing Alzheimer's disease and related dementias. But over time, we have learned that the picture is far more complicated.

For example, a group of scientists in the early 1990s announced they had identified the first genetic marker (a protein called "ApoE e4") for late-onset Alzheimer's disease, the most common form of the disease. But it was soon found that the risk level for those who carry the ApoE e4 marker is not nearly as high as in people who might inherit the rare genes associated with familial early-onset Alzheimer's disease. Even people with two copies of the ApoE e4 marker can live to old age without developing dementia. Moreover, many people with late-onset Alzheimer's disease do not have the ApoE e4 copy of the gene.[2]

This is in stark contrast to those born with genetic risk for early-onset Alzheimer's disease. A person born with one of the abnormalities associated with early onset—presenilin 1, presenilin 2, and amyloid precursor protein genes—usually develops Alzheimer's disease before the age of sixty, and he or she has a fifty-fifty chance of passing the gene along to each of his or her children. When Alzheimer's disease is caused by one of these mutations, about half the people in the family tree will develop the illness before age sixty.

Over time, experts have rejected the idea that we can identify a single genetic mutation or set of mutations as the cause of the most common form of Alzheimer's disease—that which typically shows up at age seventy-five or older. On the contrary, though we have found a number of genetic abnormalities associated with the risk of developing the disease, each is associated with only a tiny fraction of total cases. If anything, this suggests that the condition we call Alzheimer's may not be a single malady at all; in reality, there are different and perhaps very complex versions of the disease, which complicates efforts to find effective tests and treatments.

SHOULD YOU GET GENETIC TESTING FOR ALZHEIMER'S DISEASE?

Because our knowledge of the genetics of Alzheimer's is incomplete, physicians don't generally recommend genetic testing to determine a person's chances of developing the disease. Unfortunately, there is no known medical treatment to prevent, effectively slow, or stop the condition. So testing would have no practical impact on medical treatment decisions.

If, however, you're among those rare families who have cases of early-onset Alzheimer's disease in multiple generations, physicians generally recommend that you see a genetics counselor or other expert in Alzheimer's genetics. This person can advise you about testing for the inherited, early-onset form of the disease, also called "dominantly inherited Alzheimer's disease." They might also encourage you to participate in a clinical research trial exploring its genetic causes and treatments. One example is the Dominantly Inherited Alzheimer Network (DIAN; www.dian-info.org), which enrolls people who are biological adult children of a parent with a mutated gene known to cause this rare condition. Funded by the National Institute on Aging, this long-term international study aims to learn more about inherited forms of the disease so that researchers can develop screening and treatments that eventually might help all people suffering from Alzheimer's and related dementias. Coordinated by scientists at Washington University School of Medicine in St. Louis, DIAN involves fifteen research sites throughout the world, including six in the United States.

We still have much to learn in the coming years about the genetics of Alzheimer's disease and other dementias. I believe our understanding will continue to grow and change based on research using new and evolving scientific tools—especially those associated with "personalized medicine," which will use information about a person's genes, the proteins related to those genes, and environmental risk factors to prevent, diagnose, and treat illnesses. And I predict that what we call Alzheimer's disease today will be better understood, and known to be more complex than the single disease entity inferred by that single name, Alzheimer's.

STUDYING THE RIGHT PEOPLE IN THE RIGHT SETTINGS

If our progress in understanding age-related brain disease has seemed slow, there has been good reason. Looking back, I recall several studies highly touted at the time that now appear as odd detours. Mention them at scientific conferences today and you'll get blank stares; nobody recognizes or remembers them. One example: a 1987 "discovery" published in the prestigious journal *Science* that a blood abnormality called "platelet membrane fluidity" was linked to Alzheimer's disease.[3] A similar instance: a 1989 study published in *Nature* that amyloid protein deposits in blood vessels and other tissues outside the brain might be a way to detect Alzheimer's disease within it.[4] Both were promoted on the front page of national newspapers like the *New York Times* as potential breakthroughs in early diagnosis, thereby possibly capable of preventing onset and progression. But it was just a matter of time before both were shelved and forgotten.

What was the problem? The work could not be replicated in subsequent investigations among larger, more typical, and diverse community-based populations. It wasn't for lack of trying. In fact, many of the reports our team at the University of Washington and Group Health Cooperative published during that period were so-called negative studies. That is, we could not replicate others' findings in our more general, everyday population. I now believe that's because the originating research teams were studying highly specialized, small groups of self-selected patients. As our team later confirmed, these specialized populations did not resemble the general community at all. They were younger, had a stronger family history of dementia, and were more likely to carry the ApoE e4 genetic marker for Alzheimer's disease than the general population does.

In contrast, our team was conducting research among members of a large health plan. We were drawing from a community of hundreds of thousands of people who were not self-selected, and therefore provided a much more accurate picture of how Alzheimer's disease and other forms of dementia occur in everyday people living in real communities. For example, our population included far more people aged eighty-five and up. These so-called old-old people are more likely than younger folks to develop all sorts of dementia—not just the rare, more genetic-based forms of Alzheimer's disease that sometimes strike middle-aged adults.

THE HEALTHY BRAIN/HEALTHY BODY CONNECTION

Our ability to study dementia in the "real world" turned out to be an important development because it helped us discover a much stronger connection than previously realized between diseases of the brain such as Alzheimer's and the well-being of the rest of the body.

That may sound surprising some thirty years later—now that we have a much better general understanding of the way factors like physical exercise can influence our minds and emotions. In the early 1980s, however, there was a real divide among scientists pursuing knowledge on these topics. While the neuroscientists and psychiatrists focused largely on the brain and its various neurodegenerative diseases, human physiologists and non-mental-health practitioners focused on the rest of the body.

In the same way, doctors differentiated between people with Alzheimer's disease and those with so-called vascular or multi-infarct dementia, which is less common. Alzheimer's is characterized as a problem inside the brain where protein plaque and neurofibrillary tangles are believed to interfere with normal brain functions. Vascular dementia is characterized by damage to the brain from multiple small or large strokes, which involves the body's whole circulatory system—including the arteries and veins that carry blood throughout the body. Decades ago, experts assumed that a person develops just one of these causes of dementia.

All this started to change in 1985, however, when Swedish scientists studying a large population of very elderly people with dementia published a study in the *New England Journal of Medicine* showing that the proportion of those with vascular dementia was much higher than expected.[5] The study was important on several fronts. Like our work at the University of Washington and Group Health, the data came from a community-based population, not a specialized clinic, so it reflected how dementia was showing up in the real world. Also, it raised the possibility that individuals with dementia were not suffering from a single neurodegenerative process—either Alzheimer's, vascular disease, or some other discrete diagnosable illness. Rather, patients with dementia in late life might be affected by several common processes that can weaken both the brain and the rest of the body as we age. Eventually, doctors would come to call this phenomenon "mixed dementia."

Confirming the cause of a person's dementia is not easy. Imaging tests such as MRI and CT scans can provide clues to disease processes in the brain and are often used to look for uncommon causes that might mimic Alzheimer's. People can also take assessments to measure their thinking skills, physical coordination, and other possible manifestations of brainpower or weakness. But it's only after a person's death that we can definitively determine whether a person had dementia due to the pathologic changes of Alzheimer's disease. This is done by performing an autopsy and looking for telltale signs of protein plaque and neurofibrillary tangles in the brain.

Over the years, neuropathologists on our ACT research team have studied the brain tissue of hundreds of study participants following their deaths. When we first started doing the brain autopsies in 1986, our goal was simply to determine whether we had accurately diagnosed Alzheimer's disease while our study participants were still living.

But over time, the autopsies revealed that most of the people in our study with Alzheimer's disease had actually suffered from other degenerative processes in their brains as well. For example, in one study of participants averaging age eighty when first evaluated and diagnosed with dementia, we found that only thirty-four of the ninety-four cases with Alzheimer's disease at autopsy actually had "pure" Alzheimer's disease based on neuropathologic criteria. The other almost two-thirds also had signs of vascular disease or lesions associated with Parkinson's disease.[6] These findings helped us to understand that dementia due to mixed cause was far more common in very old people than either "pure" Alzheimer's disease or vascular dementia alone.

Later, when our methods for studying brains improved, we also saw that brain damage from serious head injuries, including those occurring early in life, along with conditions like heavy alcohol use, can be "mixed" in with findings of Alzheimer's disease and vascular dementia.

Other studies conducted among community-based populations in Hawaii, Chicago, and elsewhere eventually reported similar findings. And when we looked back at pioneering work by research pathologists in England and Sweden studying the brains of very old people who died in the 1950s and 1960s, we found the same results.[7]

This discovery that far more people were affected by mixed dementia than previously thought has had important implications for the way we approach screening, prevention, and treatment of dementia today. It has shifted many researchers' focus from a search for "magic bullet" causes and cures for Alzheimer's disease to an emphasis on the connection between the general health of the brain and the health of the rest of the body. It has also caused us to look for clues to dementia's causes across the whole life course.

Now that we know that large proportions of the population with dementia are suffering from forms of the condition caused (or at least complicated) by cardiovascular problems such as strokes, we also know we can prevent or delay dementia by focusing on the modifiable risk factors—that is, the things we *can* change. This includes steps we can take to prevent cardiovascular disease, such as increasing physical activity, eating a healthy diet, and not smoking. Because we know many people are suffering from dementia as a result of brain damage caused by head injuries or substance abuse, we can take preventive measures such as avoiding falls, wearing sports helmets, and addressing the overuse of drugs and alcohol. And because we now understand that factors such as good prenatal care and education can help young people develop brains resilient to stress and damage later on in life, we have yet another reason to invest in these important social infrastructures.

In short, research on Alzheimer's disease and memory problems in real-world populations over the past several decades has given us a much broader perspective on brain health and preventing dementia. We now understand there are many ways that our cognitive reserve— that is, our reservoir of brainpower—can be drained or replenished throughout our lives. And here's the real bottom line: if you want to have a healthy brain, you've got to take care of the whole body. Doing so will help you reduce your risk of developing late-life dementia and other memory problems as you age.

BRAIN HEALTH BEGINS EARLY

Protecting the brain and making it more resilient to life's stresses is a lifelong process. You can take steps at any point to shore up your thinking skills. The most important work, however, probably begins early on. We know that brain development starts in the fetus and continues throughout life, with the most intensive growth occurring prior to age six. But what can science tell us about the connection between people's early childhood experiences and their risk of developing Alzheimer's disease and dementia later on? Looking into the health of people who survived difficult socioeconomic conditions can provide clues. In fact, there's a whole body of population-based research demonstrating that socioeconomic disruptions like flu pandemics and war are linked to poor brain reserve in late life among people conceived, born, and reared during such upheavals.

During the 1990s, our research team at the University of Washington looked into this connection as well. We started by collecting county census records at the time of birth among people from two populations: those diagnosed with Alzheimer's disease and a control group the same age without the condition. The painstaking work involved finding the participants' birth counties and the conditions in those communities at the time, typically around 1900. Our conclusion? Those born in communities and families with better socioeconomic conditions had a lower chance of developing Alzheimer's disease later in life.[8] This suggests that conditions we're exposed to before birth and during early childhood can affect our likelihood of getting Alzheimer's disease *some eighty years later*.

The researchers also found that being born in suburban communities of the time versus rural areas or inner cities seemed to protect people from Alzheimer's. Those whose fathers had higher-status occupations fared better than those with low-status dads. In addition, being born to a smaller family and having an earlier rank in the birth order lowered the participants' risk. (Presumably, children's brain development benefited when the family had fewer mouths to feed and the children got relatively more parental attention.)

Getting more education early on also seems to protect the brain, although the amount of education needed is debated. One of our most fascinating studies was done in collaboration with a Taiwanese team. It involved a generation of people living on subsistence farms on a remote island off the coast of China where there were hardly any schools. The median length of formal education among the people studied was just one year. Did this lack of additional schooling affect the islanders' risk for dementia? Perhaps so. Concurrent studies of other populations where universal education is the norm showed dementia typically became more evident at age seventy, seventy-five, and beyond. But on this island near China, dementia was showing up much earlier—between ages sixty and sixty-five.[9]

Clearly, more research is needed to better understand how a child's health, education, and well-being might affect late-life brain health. But based on historic trends, I believe the outlook is good. If current trends persist, the increases in economic prosperity and universal education globally over the past century could mean reductions in worldwide rates of Alzheimer's disease and dementia in the decades to come.

LIFESTYLE AFFECTS YOUR RESERVOIR OF BRAINPOWER

Building a strong foundation of brain resilience does not end in the womb, childhood, adolescence, or early adulthood. It can continue throughout life, bolstered by habits, relationships, and a lifestyle that will help you continually replenish your cognitive reserve. The goal is not just to build a reservoir of brainpower—but also to keep filling it with resources that can last a lifetime. Factors affecting your brain reserve can include your job, your social network, and your leisure-time activities, especially physical exercise. It's not that such factors can immunize you against dementia the way a vaccine can immunize you against the measles. But making healthy lifestyle choices may increase your chances of maintaining a clearer mind over the long haul.

Regarding your work, the more intellectually challenging your job is, the lower your risk of developing dementia, and the slower your rate of cognitive decline. The relationship between job type and maintaining your brain health is complicated because influences overlap. That is, people in occupations that require lots of brainpower generally come from higher socioeconomic backgrounds and have more education. These are factors also known to protect the brain, presumably by building up your cognitive reserves. We know that the steep part of the benefit curve from both education and job complexity occurs at lower levels. So, for example, the boost a person gets from earning a high school degree would be bigger than the boost between high school graduation and a bachelor's degree. Likewise, the advantage you might gain from being a hotel reservation clerk versus a dishwasher might be more potent than the benefit of going from reservation clerk to accountant.

Many other job-related factors that contribute to physical and emotional stress may be pertinent to brain health as well—even though their long-term effects have yet to be studied. It makes sense to seek occupations that allow you to get enough leisure time and seven to eight hours of sleep each night. You want to avoid too much emotional stress, too much sitting, and too much boring, repetitious work that does not stimulate your brain and senses.

Your social life is also important for promoting healthy brain aging, avoiding dementia, and preventing a whole host of other chronic illnesses. In fact, having a supportive network of family and friends correlates with dodging early death in general. The reasons are many and complex. But basically, we need other people around to keep us talking, thinking, working, moving, caring for ourselves, and generally engaged in our lives—all necessities for good brain health.

As we'll explore in chapter 7, "Building Your Social Reserves," setting intentional goals for friendship and family relationships becomes increasingly important as you grow old. Notably, and especially in old age, it's the quality and not just the quantity of these relationships that seem most important. Our social circles naturally tend to get smaller as we age, but the last thing we want for brain health is to become socially isolated, spending too much time alone. Midlife may seem a bit early to start worrying about such things. Still, if you can imagine your days free from the daily demands of job, kids, aging parents, and so on, then you might also imagine the people who will surround you in your later years. Who will be there daily to share interesting conversations and meaningful activities? Will you have friends who inspire you to get up on your feet and out the door every day, pursuing activities that get your blood pumping and stimulate your brain? While the answers may not be clear to you today, such questions could influence your present-day goals for connecting with friends and relatives, and staying in touch with them as the years go by.

Likewise, how you spend your leisure time may impact brain health. People who pursue games like bridge or other mind-challenging pastimes appear to have better brain health than those who go into mental retirement, spending most of their days passively watching television, for instance.

One study showed how lifestyle factors like occupation and leisure activities interact; people in blue-collar jobs gained more brain protection by taking part in intellectually stimulating leisure-time activities than did college professors, perhaps because the college professors had already reached their limit of brain reserve. The blue-collar workers, on the other hand, had more room for growth, so the added leisure-time activities likely provided that extra boost.

BUT SHOULD YOU TAKE UP SUDOKU?

People often ask me if puzzles like crossword or Sudoku can help you avoid memory problems. If you saw the film *Still Alice*, you may recall how Julianne Moore's character continuously played word games, frantically hoping to drive away her symptoms of early-onset Alzheimer's. Such activities probably can't help people with problems as severe as Alice's, but they may be useful in staving off normal memory decline—and they certainly can't harm you.

I used to be skeptical about the value of so-called brain training, especially as I saw profit-driven companies increasingly promoting more games and online programs, promising to prevent age-related memory loss. Then I learned about a project called ACTIVE, started in 1998 by Sherry Willis when she was at Pennsylvania State University. Funded by the National Institute on Aging, the project aimed to prevent loss of cognitive function and promote independent living by providing seniors with a carefully constructed intervention focused on increasing reasoning, memory, and speed at processing thoughts. Her team recruited about three thousand people, average age seventy-four, in six U.S. cities, half of whom received ten training sessions followed by four booster sessions at eleven and thirty-five months.

The results, published in the *Journal of the American Medical Association* in 2006, were impressive.[10] The training had important effects on both brain performance and overall function. And the booster training produced additional value. The strongest effects seemed to be in reasoning that affected daily living—that is, abilities to complete daily tasks like meal preparation, housework, finances, telephone use, and shopping. And the researchers later showed the benefits lasted up to ten years after the program began.

This study convinced me that some brain-training activities—whether commercially produced as "games" or as part of a public-health-oriented research project—may have value. Beyond entertainment, they may actually help people gain practical skills for daily living that will serve them over time. Dr. Willis's study also convinced me that focused brain-boosting exercises can help us improve our cognitive abilities and may have some long-lasting benefits.

At the same time, such brain training has its limits. Most of the research trials show that you can improve your performance of the task you practice, but this improvement does not usually translate into a long-term benefit in other areas of cognitive performance. Also, it doesn't extend to many of the functions that deteriorate with Alzheimer's disease. So-called executive function, such as decision making and complex thinking, or the sustained ability to maintain short-term memory, does not improve.

The bottom line? For myself, I have not purchased mind-training software or programs. But I do intend to seek out brain-stimulating activities throughout my remaining years, and I counsel my patients to do the same.

PHYSICAL ACTIVITY: THE BRAIN'S BEST FRIEND

Of all the activities we can pursue to build and maintain brainpower, I believe regular physical exercise is the most potent. We know that vigorous physical activity increases blood flow to the brain, stimulates the development of brain cells and connections between them, and is linked to growth in certain critical parts of the brain. So it makes sense that reducing sitting time and increasing physical exercise can make a big difference in avoiding brain diseases such as Alzheimer's.

My first foray into research on the benefits of exercise for aging was a collaboration with University of Washington cardiologist Robert Bruce, known for developing the Bruce Protocol for the Exercise Tolerance Test, which has been used in cardiac stress testing since the 1970s. Together we wrote how regular exercise protected the body from nearly all age-related diseases and conditions, including heart disease, hypertension, depression, osteoporosis, falls, fractures, and so on. We concluded that exercise was more valuable in later life than it was in younger life, including for prevention of heart disease, which was Dr. Bruce's career-long research interest.[11] But the notion that exercise might also protect against Alzheimer's disease or other dementias seemed far-fetched at the time; all we really knew about Alzheimer's disease was that it involved the deposit of abnormal proteins in the brain. The idea of a body-mind connection affecting brain aging never occurred to us.

But over the next few decades, scientists around the world began looking in earnest at exercise—along with a whole host of lifestyle fac-tors—as a way to guard against Alzheimer's. Skepticism was common at first. For example, in 2004, Dr. Laura Fratiglioni and her colleagues at the Karolinska Institute published an evidence review of lifestyle fac-tors that might affect the risk of dementia, reporting that only half the studies to date actually showed a strong link between regular physical activity and a healthy brain.[12] (Interestingly, one study that *didn't* link reduced dementia risk to overall exercise *did* point to one form of physical activity—*dancing*—as possibly protective.[13] Evangeline Shul-er—our centenarian tango dancer introduced in chapter 1—probably missed that report. Still, her brain may have benefited from dancing's triple dose of protection: aerobic activity + social engagement + think-ing on her feet.)

So why was it so difficult for scientists to show a link between exer-cise and brain health? Because by the time people show signs of Alzhei-mer's disease, which affects memory, it's tough to document their past history of physical activity. But if you can start tracking people before they develop dementia, you can document lifestyle factors like physical activity as they age and see whether exercise makes a difference. That's what we were able to do at Group Health Cooperative and the Univer-sity of Washington with our community-based ACT study, the "living laboratory" of aging I described in chapter 1.

In a study we published in the *Annals of Internal Medicine* in 2006, we followed 1,740 Group Health members aged sixty-five and older over a six-year period.[14] Our team contacted the participants every two years to assess factors potentially affecting dementia, including exercise frequency, cognitive function, physical function, symptoms of depres-sion, and lifestyle characteristics.

After six years, 158 participants had developed dementia and 107 of those with dementia had been diagnosed with Alzheimer's disease. Peo-ple who exercised three or more times a week had a 30 to 40 percent lower risk for developing dementia compared with those who exercised fewer than three times per week. We also found that the more frail a person is, the more he or she may benefit from exercise. Even those elderly people who did modest amounts of gentle exercise, such as walking for fifteen minutes three times a week, appeared to benefit.

Our study generated a great deal of media attention—more than any other paper *Annals of Internal Medicine* had published to date, according to its editors. This was the study that put Mrs. Shuler on local television with her tango moves. It also changed the tenor of my conversations with patients about exercise. I still had no antiaging magic bullet to offer. But now I could say with absolute confidence that regular exercise is the next best thing. And over the next several months, many of my older patients took my advice to heart in ways they never had before. Those who had resisted physical activity despite other benefits—say, weight loss or preventing heart disease—suddenly added exercise to their daily routines.

I especially remember a prominent university professor who had always been deaf to my suggestions to exercise. To a very busy academic leader, his protests probably seemed rational: "Exercise takes too much time, is boring, and besides, I'm healthy enough, thank you." Indeed he did not smoke, he was not overweight, and he didn't have any age-related impairments. But then, during a checkup in his late seventies, he suddenly told me he had started taking brisk "exercise" walks as a part of his daily routine. "What changed your mind?" I asked him. "Your study of exercise and Alzheimer's disease," he responded. "I want to do everything I can to live to an old age without becoming demented."

And what about people who are already beginning to experience memory loss? Can exercise reverse the decline? An important experiment led by researchers from Australia showed in 2008 this might be the case. The team recruited 170 people over age fifty who reported they had memory problems and randomly assigned them into two groups. One was invited to develop a home-based exercise program of their choice. Most chose walking. Their task was to do 150 minutes of physical activity per week. The program was in place for six months. The other group only received information about memory loss. Cognition was measured at the end of the program and then twelve months later. Eighteen months after the program began, the exercise group had better memory and cognitive function than the information-only group.[15] In fact, the difference between the two groups was larger in this experiment than is typically seen in studies of drugs used to treat memory impairment or symptoms of memory problems. In addition, the Australian experiment, like our own 2006 study, showed that those who were the most frail benefitted the most.

This is consistent with a 2003 study led by my colleague Linda Teri at the University of Washington that showed that exercise is beneficial even after a person develops Alzheimer's. Our team randomly assigned 153 patients with Alzheimer's, along with their caregivers, to an exercise program that focused on strength, balance, and flexibility training. For about thirty minutes a day, the patients went for walks, stretched, and used light hand weights for quick exercises that they could do at home. Their caregivers were also taught a number of techniques to encourage the exercisers and to manage behavioral problems. Compared with a control group that received routine care, the patients who exercised were in better physical shape and had lower rates of depression.[16] As Dr. Teri told reporters, "These patients were much better off both physically and emotionally. They spent less time in bed and more time being active. The intervention really changed their day-to-day functions and improved their mood. Over all, they were happier."[17]

Meanwhile, I've seen the difference among patients with Alzheimer's in my own medical practice. For many, exercise seems to mitigate their symptoms and slow their rate of their decline. It's not a panacea, erasing the effects of the disease, but it gives people more time, allowing them to live fuller lives before they reach late-stage dementia. And by staying stronger and being able to get around safely, they avoid becoming bed- and chair-bound until as late as possible in the course of the disease. They can have a more meaningful and fuller life—even as they suffer memory loss and other problems of Alzheimer's.

Correlation between physical activity and the mind—even among those already affected by dementia—is further evidence of the way the mind and the body are inextricably linked. To care for your mind, you must care for the whole body.

PROTECTING YOUR BRAIN FROM INJURY AND OTHER RISKS

While physical activity helps you to build new brainpower, there's much you can do to save what you've accumulated—an effort that becomes increasingly important with age. As the aging brain changes naturally over time, it becomes more susceptible to harm. Here are some practical ways to protect your brain from some of life's common hazards:

Avoid head injury: Evidence is mounting that sport-related head injuries may contribute to dementia later in life. The media have focused on football players who develop dementia relatively early after multiple concussions, but concussions can happen in many ways at any stage in life and can result in cumulative damage to the brain. In studying the brain tissue of ACT study participants following their deaths, we've found that traumatic brain injuries don't cause the same kind of damage as that seen in Alzheimer's disease. But it is a degenerative form of brain damage. Head injuries that result in concussion can result in cognitive problems—especially for aging brains.

Bottom line: Avoid head injuries caused by sports, falls, traffic accidents, domestic violence, or other trauma at all stages of life. Do all you can to keep your head safe from bumps and bruises. This includes wearing a helmet when biking, skiing, or participating in other sports. (Chapter 6, "Building Your Physical Reserves: Your Bones, Muscles, Heart, Vision, and Hearing," provides practical information on how to avoid falls, the most common cause of head injuries among older people.)

Moderate or avoid alcohol consumption: Expert opinion is mixed on how moderate alcohol consumption affects brain health, but we know that long-term overuse is clearly harmful, leading to cognitive impairment. That's just one of many good reasons to limit your drinking as you age. (Moderate drinking is defined as one drink per day for women and two drinks per day for men.) Keep in mind that older people typically feel alcohol's effects more than younger people do. This can lead to falls and other accidents due to impaired balance and judgment. Also, drinking can make other health problems worse, and it can interfere with prescription drugs you may be taking for chronic illness.

Be mindful of the drugs you take: Talk with your primary care doctor often about your medicine—both prescription and nonprescription. For brain health, you want to avoid dangerous interactions and overmedicating, issues that can cause memory problems and dementia. Try to stay informed about possible long-term side effects of drugs you take for chronic conditions.

For example, our research discovered in 2015 that a class of drugs called anticholinergics, which includes certain common antidepressants, bladder drugs, and antihistamines, are linked to a slightly higher chance of developing dementia.[18] This includes the drug chlorpheniramine, an antihistamine found in many popular over-the-counter sleeping aids and allergy and cold remedies. This research convinced me that, in general, you should try to avoid this class of drugs.

Benzodiazepines are also notorious for harming brain function. These are sedatives commonly prescribed for insomnia or anxiety. And while our research determined that benzodiazepines are not linked to dementia, they are bad for older people because they can cause confusion, sleepiness, and loss of balance, leading to falls and fractures.

What should you do if you're an older person whose doctor prescribes drugs known to impair brain function? I recommend that you voice your concerns and then weigh the pros and cons of taking it based on your individual situation. As researchers discover more about drug safety in the elderly, questions like these will continue to surface. (See more on drug safety in chapter 6.)

Control your risk for heart problems: Cardiovascular risks—including hypertension (high blood pressure), high cholesterol, diabetes, and atrial fibrillation—can raise your risk for Alzheimer's disease and dementia as well. So do what you can to control such conditions with a healthy diet and exercise. Don't smoke. And if your doctor recommends medications such as blood-pressure-lowering drugs, statins for control of high cholesterol, or antidiabetic medications, take them as prescribed.

Avoid a high-sugar diet: Research has long shown that high blood sugar due to diabetes can increase your risk for many health problems, including Alzheimer's disease and other dementias. But more recently, our team discovered that high blood sugar raises your risk for these conditions even in people *without* diabetes.[19] This discovery gives you one more reason to avoid food and drinks high in sugar, such as sweetened sodas and other high-fructose beverages. And although diet fads may seem to come and go, it's helpful to know that consensus has been growing for many years in favor of the Mediterranean diet and the DASH diet to preserve brain health. Both emphasize fruits, vegetables, whole grains, only healthy fats, and limited amounts of red meat and salt.

Limit stress: As we discussed in chapter 3, "Acceptance: Discovering Aging on Its Own Terms," older bodies can have a harder time adapting to change and other stressors. One reason is that cortisol, a hormone secreted when you're under stress, has a stronger effect on older brains, challenging your ability to recover from emotional upset. Knowing this, it's best to take change slowly and learn ways to cope with anxiety or tension.

Sleep well: Research has shown that inadequate sleep is associated with slower thinking and risk of dementia. While individual needs vary greatly—especially as we age—most guidelines recommend getting seven to nine hours of sleep a night. Frequent trouble sleeping does not mean you need to take sleeping pills for insomnia. Such drugs can actually make cognitive problems worse. You may simply need to improve your "sleep hygiene" by developing habits that help your body settle down at night. (Examples: Avoid caffeine late in the day. Don't use your computer or smart phone in bed. Make your room cool, dark, and quiet.) Problems sleeping may also be related to sleep apnea, a common breathing disorder that interferes with sleep and can be treated without drugs.

GAINING YEARS OF QUALITY LIFE

Reviewing the growing bounty of evidence that our brains can continue to grow and change throughout our lives, I feel optimistic that we can protect and build our brainpower for a better experience growing old.

We can't expect to keep our minds forever young. Eventually, everybody experiences some loss of memory and cognitive function with age. Like any part of the body, your brain experiences wear and tear. And there's certainly nothing you can do about past experiences that already may have stacked the brain-reserve deck against you (i.e., playing youth football or taking harmful drugs over a long period of time).

But you can take steps today to prevent harmful brain injuries and illness while maintaining healthy habits like exercise and an active social life. By doing so, you can minimize the depletion of your brain reserve while adding more power to the reservoir for a net gain of healthy years.

I think of my own father in this regard, a warmhearted, sociable man who grew up during the hard times of the Great Depression in a farming community in South Dakota. Although he did not get to complete college, he had a rewarding career as an insurance salesman, a strong marriage, and a happy family life. I have many wonderful memories of my childhood growing up outside of Portland, Oregon, colored by my father's boundless enthusiasm for home crafts and projects. He had my sister and me raising rabbits, growing vegetables and fruit trees, and harvesting more apples than we could possibly cook into pies, cobblers, and applesauce. He was also a master weaver, supplying our home and church with beautiful Norwegian linens and rugs.

His life was not always easy, however, and some of his troubles likely took a toll on his brain. He suffered a head injury in a bad car accident when he was in his seventies. He also had a bout of clinical depression for which he received electroshock therapy, which was standard treatment in the late 1960s. Still, he came through this period with his spirits and intellect intact. In retirement, he spent winters living "off the grid" in Arizona with my mom, where he made new friends, knotted rugs, tended to a cactus garden, and took long walks down desert roads in a quirky neighborhood called Javelina Flats. During the rest of the year, they lived in our family's original community near Portland, where he took a three-mile walk each day, often to a local coffee shop for long conversations with old and new friends.

All that exercise kept my dad's heart generally healthy, but by his mideighties I could see that his memory was starting to slip. My mom was also becoming more frail. After much discussion (and resistance to moving from their family home of more than fifty years), they finally decided to move into a senior-living community called Rose Villa. Residents could live independently in individual units, or if they needed a bit of extra help, they could get that too. The community also had a wonderful health center for residents who became disabled and needed continual care.

My parents moved into a duplex apartment where they lived independently at first. But because of my father's background—his head injury and electroshock therapy in particular—I expected he would soon develop full-blown dementia and require the higher level of care that the health center offered. Fortunately, I was proven wrong; there were things about my father I had not taken into account—his gregarious personality, his determination to stay active, and his interest in helping others, especially those who were confined to bed, lonely, or a bit confused themselves.

Soon after Mom and Dad moved into Rose Villa, Dad discovered the health center, albeit in a much different manner than I expected. Virtually every morning he would walk to the center, cheerfully greet the staff, and then make his "rounds," visiting each resident—whether they were able to respond or not—with his characteristic salute, "Hi, Sunshine!" After that, he headed out for a three-mile walk around the grounds. He continued this routine religiously for about eight years, lifting the spirits of staff and residents. This joyous daily trek also lifted his spirits, and I think it gave meaning to his later years.

It was not until age ninety-five that my father's dementia became so serious that he had to move into the health center. In the meantime, he had what I never would have predicted at this age: eight years of quality life, living independently with my mother in their own apartment. Once he moved to the health center and adjusted, he seemed happy, saying both hello and good-bye to his visiting grandsons with one simple phrase: "Keep smiling."

He passed away eighteen months later at age ninety-seven. I had been doing research on Alzheimer's disease for nearly thirty years by the time my father died. And yet his experience gave me a perspective on brain health I found both surprising and inspirational.

But the brain health story is certainly not the whole story on enlightened aging. We can also take action to build physical and social reserves.

6

BUILDING YOUR PHYSICAL RESERVES
Your Bones, Muscles, Heart, Vision, and Hearing

When my mother was in her late fifties, she had a series of mishaps, beginning with a fall at an outdoor wedding in Montana. Her heel got caught in a gopher hole and down she went, breaking her ankle. Over the next five years she suffered five more broken bones related to falls—fractures of her hip, wrist, elbow, and each kneecap.

I arranged for her to see an endocrinologist who confirmed our suspicions: my mother had developed osteoporosis, which means "porous bones" in Greek. The condition increases your risk of fractures, in some cases leading to crippling disability. After age sixty-five, it affects about one in four women and one in twenty men, and frequency increases with age. My mom developed it relatively young, perhaps because of her early menopause, which puts some women at an even higher risk.

Mom's doctor prescribed various drug treatments advocated at the time. Most of them caused unpleasant side effects and had to be stopped. (The exceptions were calcium, vitamin D, and estrogen, which she continued for many years.)

But here's the interesting part: the doctor also recommended that my mom start exercising every day. Up to that point, she had never been physically active. Although she grew up on a ranch in Montana, she hadn't done much manual labor. And like many women her age, she had never played sports nor exercised for fun. She was trained as a lab tech and later a librarian, so her jobs outside the home were always sedentary. But in middle age, she heeded her doctor's advice and started a routine of daily walking and leg-strengthening exercises. After that, the frequent fractures stopped.

It wasn't that physical activity "cured" my mother's osteoporosis. There's evidence that weight-bearing exercise can build bone mass, but by the time my mother started her walking program, her effort was probably too little, too late for that effect. In fact, periodic scans and x-rays showed that her bones continued to get thinner as she aged. Her estrogen, vitamin D, and calcium supplements may have lessened the decline, but osteoporosis is a progressive condition.

So why, after so many fractures, did she stop breaking bones? She stopped falling, thanks to exercise that increased her muscle strength and balance. So instead of suffering the kinds of fractures that spell the end of an active life for so many older people, she had three more decades to spend gardening, traveling, and strolling with my dad in the Arizona sunset.

My mother lived to age ninety-seven. And eventually, progressive osteoporosis and degenerative arthritis did cause her bones and muscles to decline. The last two years of her life she needed a wheelchair and assistance. But I am quite certain that she would have become disabled earlier if she had not started walking regularly in middle age. Instead, she surprised us by going decades with no further fractures. She still had the underlying condition of osteoporosis, which no "magic bullet" could cure. But she found the next best thing: exercise!

My mother's story holds an important lesson for those who may wonder, is it ever too late to start building physical reserves for a resilient old age? Absolutely not. At whatever age you begin, you're very likely to see positive results. For my mom, the most obvious advantage was that she stopped breaking bones when she stopped falling. But her proactive approach probably helped her build reserves in other areas too—such as her brainpower and heart health—all of which helped her to stay well and independent as she grew old.

Keep in mind that your chances of postponing disability until very late in life largely depend on four interrelated functions: your abilities to think, move, hear, and see. In the previous chapter, we explored building and maintaining mental reserves through brain health. In this chapter, you'll learn ways to grow reserves for physical resilience as well. This includes a healthy musculoskeletal system, cardiovascular system, hearing, and vision.

As with the brain, it *is* possible to slow the rate of aging-related physical decline in these parts of your body—and, in some cases, even reverse it. The key is to approach aging mindfully, accumulating and protecting your physical resources as much as possible. Doing so will give you a greater well to draw from—whether you're struck by sudden illness or simply experience the decline that naturally occurs over time.

BUILDING A HEALTHY FRAMEWORK: BONES, MUSCLES, AND JOINTS

As my mother's story illustrates, the health of our musculoskeletal system is important to our entire experience of well-being. It's helpful to think of our bones, joints, and muscles as a single unit, a framework that supports almost everything we do in life. We need this structure to work well so we can get around our homes and our communities, keep ourselves active, safe, and well cared for. It also helps us do what's needed to keep the brain and heart healthy, such as exercising and staying socially active.

In youth, most of us take the health of our bones, muscles, and joints for granted until we're injured. We may grumble about the temporary inconvenience of a cast or crutches. But once we heal from that broken bone or pulled muscle, we forget about our injuries because our mobility and independence are restored.

By middle age, however, many begin to imagine how living with chronic conditions like osteoarthritis or osteoporosis could affect well-being in old age. For some people, such conditions start slowly, almost without notice. They may feel a little stiffness or an occasional ache, and chalk it up to "just getting old." But as the pain increasingly interferes with work and pleasure, it can no longer be ignored. Treatment can range from over-the-counter pain relievers, to alternative therapies like yoga or massage, to surgery for fractures or worn-out joints. And in serious cases, long-term loss of function and mobility may result.

Can age-related musculoskeletal problems be prevented? To a certain degree, yes. But as with memory loss and aging, we can expect some degeneration in our bones, muscles, and joints over time. That's why it's so important to do all we can to build up our reserves of bone and muscle strength while we can, and to prevent unnecessary "wear and tear" whenever possible. Currently, about half of all people aged ninety and older are functionally disabled by some form of degeneration to their musculoskeletal system. I believe that by the time the boomer generation reaches that age, that number will be smaller. Just as our society is increasingly staving off mental decline until very old age, we may soon be able to do the same with physical decline.

MAINTAINING BONE TO AVOID FRACTURES

Osteoporosis is a gradual loss of the mineral matrix that gives your bones strength and resistance. We build up the mineral content in our bones when we're young, reaching a peak in our thirties. (Weight-bearing exercise is one way to strengthen bones during this process, so it's especially important for young women, who are at higher risk for osteoporosis than men, to get plenty of physical activity.)

But as we age, we slowly lose bone density. For women, this loss typically intensifies at menopause as estrogen levels decrease. For men, bone density starts to decline about a decade later.

If you have osteoporosis, bone loss happens much earlier and faster than usual. A person is considered to have osteoporosis if their bone-mineral density is below the level that 95 percent of people have at peak density. By this definition, women over the age of seventy-five are twice as likely to have osteoporosis as men the same age.

Osteoporosis doesn't usually cause symptoms itself. Rather, it results in fractures—often a broken hip, wrist, or rib caused by a fall or even a minor accident. Often osteoporosis is first suspected when a person suffers a fracture from a mishap not likely to break a healthy bone—say, bumping into furniture or lifting a heavy package.

People with osteoporosis may also develop a curvature of the upper spine, just below the neck, commonly called "dowager's hump." This happens as gravity causes the vertebrae in the upper spine to spontaneously collapse and wedge together. The severity of the curve and associated pain can vary from barely noticeable to severe.

Earlier in your senior years—say, in your sixties, seventies, or even early eighties—osteoporotic fractures might result in pain, immobility, hospitalizations, surgery, or placement in a rehabilitation center to heal. But later on, some fractures can be life threatening. For example, a hip fracture can ultimately result in a fatal outcome because of difficulty healing and complications that result when a person is bedridden.

Two different types of medications are typically prescribed to stop or even reverse bone-mineral loss after a person has a fracture due to weak bones. One is the hormone supplement estrogen, which women may use after menopause, although it is known to increase the risk of cardio-vascular health problems and certain kinds of cancer. The other is a class of drugs call bisphosphonates. (Examples are alendronate, which has the brand name Fosamax, and ibandronate, brand named Boniva.) Bisphosphonates increase bone density and reduce fracture risk, but sometimes they make the bone more brittle. They have been known to cause spontaneous jaw fractures after prolonged use. Also, they can cause serious heartburn, leading to damage of the lower esophagus. For these reasons, some people can't tolerate this class of drugs.

Because both drug types have such serious side effects, I always have a careful conversation with my patients about risks and benefits before prescribing either. And I generally don't recommend that anybody take these drugs for longer than about ten years.

THE BEST PROTECTION: PREVENT FALLS!

I also have serious discussions with all my older patients—whether or not they have osteoporosis—about ways to prevent falling, which often leads to serious fractures. Studies show that each year one-third of Americans over sixty-five take a fall, making it the leading cause of both fatal and nonfatal injuries among older adults. More than 95 percent of hip fractures are caused by falls.

These commonsense measures can reduce your risk:

Stay physically active: Even a simple exercise like daily walking, swimming, or bicycling can help tremendously by building muscle strength and reducing fatigue. Add activities to increase balance and you'll be even better off. Balance is often a focus of exercise classes tailored to seniors. It's also an important element in yoga, Pilates, and tai chi, the ancient Chinese practice of continuous, controlled, and slow movement to improve physical and mental well-being. One study published decades ago showed that people who practiced tai chi dramatically improved their balance and prevention of falls compared to people who did not do the practice. These benefits have since been validated in other studies.[1]

If illness or injury slows you down, make rehabilitation exercises a top priority. The overall fitness you'll gain can help you prevent falling, and if you do fall, you'll suffer less injury and recover faster.

Wear proper shoes or slippers: A team affiliated with our ACT study did research to determine whether falls happen more often from slipping or tripping—and what kind of footwear could best prevent a tumble.[2] We asked several hundred participants to keep journals, reporting what they were wearing on their feet each time they fell. Then we examined their shoe and floor surfaces to determine how much friction was present. (One energetic participant—an avid skier—called us each time he fell on the slopes, but we decided to record his data one time only!)

The results of the study were striking. We learned the following:

- Most falls are caused by slipping, not tripping.
- The safest shoes have laces or Velcro fasteners, adequate heel support, and nonslip soles. (Translation: wear a good tennis shoe.)
- The highest risk comes from walking around barefoot or in stocking feet—even indoors.

I also recommend avoiding high heels.

The data from this study was so striking that research staff at the consumer advocacy group Public Citizen urged the U.S. Secretary of Health and Human Services to send a reminder with every Social Security check: "Seniors, be safe! Do not go barefoot or walk about in your stocking feet!"

Check your medications—especially sleeping pills: Talk to your doctor if you're experiencing dizziness or fatigue. The problem might be alleviated by stopping or lowering dosages on certain medications. Drugs for high blood pressure and chronic pain often cause balance problems, leading to falls. Also implicated in falls are antidepressants, antipsychotics, and antianxiety and sleeping medications—especially benzodiazepine tranquilizers.[3] Sleeping medications are a particular problem. As I've sometimes told my patients, "Nobody ever died because they could not sleep, but I've seen people who broke their hips because their sleeping pills made them wobbly."

Get the right equipment: Use canes or walkers, if you need them. And if you fall frequently, consider wearing hip pads to prevent fractures.

Be safe in the bathroom: Many falls happen around the toilet, bathtub, and shower. So install and use handholds. Get a shower chair if you're unsteady standing for long periods. Keep a pair of slippers beside your bed to wear when nature calls. And gentlemen, consider sitting down to urinate—especially during the night. A condition called "micturition syncope" sometimes causes older men to have a sudden drop in blood pressure when they are urinating, particularly just after waking. This can cause fainting and a fall. But you're less likely to fall if you're seated.

Avoid too much alcohol: Pace your drinking to avoid tipsiness. Also beware of interactions between your drinks and prescription medications that might make you unsteady.

Eliminate household hazards: Get rid of loose electrical cords and throw rugs in your home. Avoid slippery floors and icy surfaces. Make sure rooms and passageways are well lit. Use night-lights.

Take vitamin D: Several studies show that people who take vitamin D supplements have improved muscle strength, better balance, and reduced falls. This may be especially important for people living in high northern latitudes where absence of sunlight during the short days of winter reduces the body's ability to use vitamin D to maintain bone strength, thereby contributing to more osteoporosis.

STRONG MUSCLES KEEP US GOING

My mother's story shows the importance of building muscle strength through regular exercise, even though her medical diagnosis—osteoporosis—was a condition of the bones. Without strong muscles, you can't do the work needed to keep the entire body safe and strong. This is true for whatever health goal you want to pursue or malady you're trying to prevent.

Like so many changes that occur with aging, the size and strength of your muscles naturally declines over time—especially if you don't use them. So by the time people reach their eighties or so, many are no longer strong enough to perform some very basic functions, and their weakness may be a sign of trouble ahead. For example, they can't stand up from a seated position without pushing off of the chair with their arms. Once you become too weak to do this, you may be at higher risk for falling and other injuries that can be disabling and interfere with your ability to live independently. And just as astronauts quickly lose muscle function when weightless, people in old age who "take to bed" or spend their entire days in an easy chair experience rapid decline in physical function.

But loss of muscle strength is not inevitable if you're willing to take action. In fact, research shows you can build muscle at any age, as long as you can be physically active.

A research team from Tufts University opened my eyes to this possibility with a study they published in the *Journal of the American Medical Association* in 1990. It involved ten people, ages eighty-six to ninety-six, living in a long-term care facility in Boston. Although all were able to walk, eight had a history of falls and seven used either a walker or cane for balance.

The research team designed an intervention to improve this. They met with the participants three times a week, leading them through a series of resistance exercises to build strength in their quadriceps and hamstrings, large muscles in the back and front of the upper leg. After eight weeks, the results were remarkable. The participants showed dramatic gains in muscle strength. Two participants no longer needed their canes, and one person who previously could not easily move from sitting to standing was now able to do so. CT scans showed that muscle mass in their legs had improved significantly.

The researchers wrote, "Because muscle strength decreases by 30 percent to 40 percent during the course of adult lifespan, it is likely that these subjects were stronger than they had been in many years previously."[4]

But what happened when the program ended? After four weeks of no more training, the elderly participants' leg strength declined by 32 percent. Everyday sedentary living was taking them back to where they started. This study—and many others that followed—showed that old people can indeed gain strength through exercise, *even in their nineties.*

But in order to maintain that strength, they have to keep exercising. If they don't, they'll soon lose the ground they gained.

A WAKE-UP CALL

Years later, I watched one of my patients use this phenomenon to her very best advantage. Laura was a retired physician in her midseventies with a passion for good food and travel, but little interest in fitness. Anytime I suggested that she try to get more physical activity into her routine, she seemed uninterested. Hers was "a life of the mind." She had no time for exercise.

Laura's visits were infrequent; she came to see me only when she was preparing for a long trip to some exotic locale. This time, she would be going with her daughter, a frequent traveling companion. Given Laura's age, the pair wanted to know if I thought the trip was a good idea.

But when I saw them walk down the hall in the clinic, I was shocked by how slowly Laura was moving. It had been over a year since our last visit, and she was clearly in decline. Once in the exam room, Laura and her daughter chatted excitedly about their upcoming journey. I did a physical exam and we reviewed Laura's vital signs and lab tests. There were no apparent signs of trouble. Still, I could tell that her daughter was concerned.

Laura was seated in a chair next to me. I asked her if she could stand without using her arms for support. She hesitated for a moment and then leaned forward, giving it a try. "I can't believe I can't do this," she said, annoyed. She lurched forward again, gaining momentum, but still she could not lift herself out of the chair. The only way she could stand was to vigorously push herself off the chair using her hands and arms.

That's when I knew it wasn't safe for Laura to travel. And though it was difficult, I tried to be completely honest with her. I explained that her inability to do this simple move was an indication of how weak she had become. And unless she could get stronger, she would be at risk for falls and serious injury—something she would not want to happen anywhere, much less in a foreign country.

I also told her it was entirely possible that she could make the trip later on. But she would need to become much stronger. And unless she took action to do so, she might soon be unable to do much of anything independently, let alone resume her travels. I recommended that she pursue strength training, focusing on major muscle groups. Her goals would be to restore and maintain her ability to lift herself up and walk more steadily. I knew that with persistent strengthening exercises, she would be able to build up her leg muscles just as the participants in the Tufts University study had done.

Fortunately, Laura accepted my recommendation. Instead of making that trip with her daughter, she contacted a spa-type center that specializes in rehabilitation and strength training for older people and those with chronic illness. With supervised training, she developed a routine that she learned to do on her own. And most importantly, she stayed motivated to maintain her progress once she got back to Seattle.

When I saw Laura about six months later, she walked through the clinic at a considerably faster pace. Once in the exam room, she proudly showed me that she could stand up from a chair without using her arms. And then she told me about the next trip she was planning to take with her daughter.

I was so glad Laura had used our last visit as her wake-up call to change her sedentary habits and to finally begin exercising. But I also wondered how I might have inspired her to begin sooner. Ideally, enlightened agers will have the foresight to establish routines early and maintain their physical reserves over time.

PROTECT YOUR JOINTS TOO!

Like many in my generation, I used to love running. In fact, I was a cross-country runner in high school and enjoyed jogging well into my forties. But by the time I reached fifty I had to face the cruel truth of human anatomy: the cartilage on the ends of our bones wears out over time—a condition called degenerative joint disease or osteoarthritis. This, along with the damage I did to my knees while skiing and climbing, meant my running days were over. I decided that if I was going to stay fit, I'd have to find a new way to exercise.

It's a common story, especially as boomers hit middle age and start to feel the impact (literally) of all their previous physical activity. They're especially noticing it in their knees, shoulders, backs, wrists, and fingers, places that have borne a lot of pressure over the years. How people adapt to problem joints can have a significant effect on their quality of life in later years. Fortunately, advances now allow seniors to maintain function despite serious joint problems. Progress ranges from education about preserving aging joints and range of motion, to improved medications, to joint replacement surgery.

Here are two things you can do to keep your joints healthy:

1. Have a regular exercise regime designed to build muscles around your joints. This may involve some strength training every other day. The exercises should provide resistance without causing joint pain. Some people use hand weights, exercise bands, or weight machines. It's usually best to learn about this in an exercise class or from a trainer or physical therapist so you can do the exercises safely. Activities such as bicycling, water aerobics, yoga, and Pilates may also help you build strength around joints, along with "core strength" for your torso.

2. Don't overuse joints once they start to become painful. You'll want to keep exercising, but doing so in ways that take the stress off painful areas. Swimming can be great for this. Also, like me, many people have to avoid exercise that jars their joints, such as running. Switch to walking, bicycling, or swimming instead.

USE PAIN MEDICATION CAUTIOUSLY: NSAIDS AND ACETAMINOPHEN

Our knowledge about medications for joint pain continues to evolve. Osteoarthritis causes joints to feel swollen, warm, and painful. Aspirin used to be the mainstay for treating such inflammation, but side effects—especially heartburn and other stomach problems—are common with aspirin. Today, doctors generally recommend judicious use of other nonsteroidal anti-inflammatory drugs (NSAIDs) such as ibuprofen (brand names Advil or Motrin) and naproxen (brand name Aleve) because these alternatives are not as hard on the stomach as aspirin. But you should be cautious, taking NSAIDs only as directed. Overuse can cause serious side effects—including bleeding and ulcers in the stomach and colon; heartburn, inflammation, and bleeding in the esophagus;

and kidney problems leading to kidney failure and elevated blood pressure. NSAIDs' hazardous side effects are more common for older people and those who use the drugs regularly at high doses over a long period of time.

Surprisingly, the pain reliever acetaminophen (brand name Tylenol) is a good choice for many people. Although it's not an anti-inflammatory, it does provide effective pain relief and is much safer than many other medications.

Avoid taking narcotic (also called opioid) pain relievers for osteoarthritis. These include drugs such as hydrocodone (brand names include Lorcet or Vicodin) and oxycodone (brand names include OxyContin or Percocet). These drugs are not very effective for long-term use, can cause side effects, and are highly addictive. Also, older people using them commonly experience problems with balance and thinking. Their long-term use for noncancer pain has been linked to increased hospitalizations and deaths from accidental overdose.

Alternatives to pain medication like massage, physical therapy routines, acupuncture, and meditation can help people with joint pain and don't have the side effects of prescription drugs.

Mostly, I encourage patients with joint issues to stay active. Combining basic aerobic activity with strength training, stretching, and range-of-motion exercises can help you to minimize the effects that aging joints can have on quality of life. Medications can be helpful, but physical activity is more so.

LESSONS FROM OUR RESEARCH ON BACK PAIN

The power of exercise to address chronic pain is clear to me when I think about the way care for back pain has evolved over the last few decades. As I mentioned in chapter 2 in relation to overuse of x-rays, doctors approached back pain much differently in the past, focusing first on whether patients needed specialized tests and eventually surgery. For acute back pain, long-term bed rest and narcotic medications were often prescribed.

But now we know that just the opposite approach is better. Research has shown that early surgery for back pain is unwise, acute back pain typically gets better within a few days or weeks, and bed rest usually results in worse outcomes. In most cases, it's far better for people with uncomplicated back pain (that is, pain without a specific cause like cancer or a fracture) to stay active. Physical therapy programs promote better range of motion and core strength, reducing acute back problems for most people. And when back pain is chronic, the ancient Asian practice of yoga—probably an evolutionary adaptation to a common physical problem—is remarkably effective. In fact, my colleagues Daniel Cherkin and Karen Sherman at Group Health Research Institute have studied yoga,[5] massage,[6] acupuncture,[7] chiropractic care, and mindfulness-based stress reduction[8] for treatment of back pain and found that all of these nondrug treatments work well.

I believe Western medicine's mistake in the past has been to "medicalize" common back pain—that is, to treat this highly prevalent and variable condition as though it were a disease to cure with bed rest, medication, and surgery. Instead, back pain can be seen as a basic human condition, a normal part of life. Understanding this, we now know that activity—including rehabilitative exercises and alternative approaches such as yoga—is often a much better course.

JOINT REPLACEMENT SURGERY—WHEN THE TIME IS RIGHT

At the same time, we can't ignore the benefits of one high-tech advance in recent decades: the development of surgery to replace joints worn out by osteoarthritis. Such operations are helping millions of seniors avoid severe disability and pain with aging. In fact, Dr. John Charnley, the pioneering surgeon who developed total hip replacement, received the Albert Lasker Award (sometimes referred to as America's Nobel Prize) in 1974, honoring him for improving millions of lives. Hip and knee replacements have become much safer and more effective in recent years and are now among the most common surgeries for older people.

An activated patient considering joint replacement will want to be aware of two important issues:

1. *Timing:* When to have a hip or knee replaced is an important question to discuss with your physician. The benefits of replace-

ment don't last forever. So if you're fairly young, you may decide to wait so that you don't need a second replacement later on. Research shows that patients undergoing second operations often have more complications and side effects. On the other hand, you don't want to wait too long because the muscles surrounding your joints are probably becoming weaker as time goes by. This could make your rehabilitation lengthier. Also, the longer you wait, the fewer years you'll have to enjoy the benefit of the operation.

2. *Do "prehab" in addition to rehab:* Health care organizations have developed extensive rehabilitation programs to help patients recover following joint replacement surgery, and that's important. But your strength and fitness prior to surgery can also have an important effect on the outcome. Sometimes people are so weak and frail going into the operation that they can't benefit from the operation. To ensure that you get the most out of joint replacement, try to be as physically fit as possible beforehand. Prehab work should address general fitness through non-weight-bearing aerobic exercise such as cycling or swimming. Your doctor might also recommend focused muscle strengthening, such as isometric exercises.

BUILDING YOUR CARDIOVASCULAR HEALTH

Your heart and blood vessels are the mechanisms that deliver oxygen and other nutrients to all your body's vital organs and tissues. So it's little wonder that the health of your cardiovascular system has a huge effect on your functional well-being, quality of life, and survival.

Medical science has discovered a tremendous amount about the risk and treatment of cardiovascular disease over the past fifty years. As a result, deaths from heart attacks and strokes in the United States have decreased significantly.

Meanwhile, however, obesity has contributed to a greater prevalence of many chronic cardiovascular-related diseases. This means many more people are now living into old age with cardiovascular conditions such as atherosclerosis (hardening of the arteries), hypertension (high blood pressure), diabetes, and more. And many are living with the discomfort and disability that such conditions bring—problems like fatigue, shortness of breath, chest pain, impaired mobility, depression, dementia, and so on.

But here's the good news emerging from research on the overlap between cardiovascular health and healthy aging: for most people, such suffering does *not* have to be the norm! Yes, genetics plays a part, and there's nothing you can do about inheriting a risk for heart disease from your parents. But cardiovascular risk is related to lifestyle as well. That means you have a remarkable opportunity to prevent heart and blood vessel problems as you age.

Many people can reduce their chances of cardiovascular disease and its ill effects if they practice these five health habits:

1. Don't smoke.
2. Exercise regularly.
3. Eat a healthy diet.
4. Maintain a healthy weight.
5. Manage your stress.

Also, there are many effective medications for treating cardiovascular disease if healthy habits alone are not enough.

Granted, some people follow all the best health advice and still develop heart conditions because of their inherited risk or just plain, old-fashioned bad luck. That's unfortunate, but certainly no reason to abandon lifestyle-related efforts to stay well. Evidence shows that healthy habits are always worthwhile because they can keep the worst effects of cardiovascular disease (and other health problems) at bay while bolstering the effect of life-saving treatments.

TWO BIG PROBLEMS TO AVOID: ATHEROSCLEROSIS AND HYPERTENSION

One of the most common cardiovascular problems is atherosclerosis, also called coronary artery disease or "hardening of the arteries." It's related to hypertension, which can be both a cause and a result of atherosclerosis.

When you have atherosclerosis, a waxy substance called plaque builds up inside arteries in your heart and elsewhere, making it difficult for blood vessels to carry oxygen-rich blood to your heart and other areas of the body, including your brain. Plaque consists of fats called triglycerides, along with cholesterol, calcium, and other material, such as small bits of clotted blood. When plaque blocks the flow of blood to your heart, it can cause a heart attack or other damage, such as heart arrhythmias or congestive heart failure. Plaques can also rupture and cause damage. If plaque blocks the flow of blood to your brain, it can cause a stroke or other brain-related problems such as a transient is-chemic attack (TIA) or mini-stroke, resulting in cognitive problems or the kind of vascular dementia I mentioned in chapter 5. Many other problems can result from atherosclerosis as well, including kidney prob-lems, eye problems—even erectile dysfunction.

Atherosclerosis can be caused by many different factors that damage the inside of your arteries. These include smoking, inflammation, high levels of sugar in your blood from diabetes, or high levels of LDL ("bad") cholesterol in your blood. It can also be caused by hyperten-sion—that is, blood flowing through your arteries at a pressure higher than normal.

Atherosclerosis often runs in families. You're considered to have this risk if your father or brother is diagnosed before age fifty-five or your mother or sister is diagnosed before age sixty-five. Hypertension can also be inherited. The risk of both conditions increases dramatically with age. But healthy lifestyle choices minimize your chances of being affected. Also, you can be mindful about the medications you take—and avoid. Certain prescription drugs for asthma or hormone treatment, for example, can raise your blood pressure; so if you take such drugs and have high blood pressure, you should discuss the potential risks with your doctor.

Once you've been diagnosed with hypertension, your doctor may encourage you to check your blood pressure regularly and track the results. Tracking can help you see how lifestyle factors and medication are affecting your levels and what you can do to keep your blood pres-sure at a level that's healthy for you.

Guidelines for healthy blood pressure levels change from time to time. In recent years some experts have called for more aggressive lowering of blood pressure. Some, for example, recommend that people age fifty and older aim for a target of less than 120 millimeters of mercury (mmHg) rather than 130, which was the standard in the past.

In fact, a landmark research study called SPRINT[9] was published in the *New England Journal of Medicine* in 2015 calling for 120. Meanwhile, some other studies showed this may be too low for certain elderly people, putting them at risk for fainting, kidney problems, faster cognitive decline, and higher mortality. Stay tuned, as this is an area where medical advice is changing.

I believe that patients need to get personalized advice from their doctors regarding the blood pressure level that's best for them as individuals. The most important thing is to be aware that high blood pressure can be a risk, so you want to keep it at a reasonably low level. But you don't want your blood pressure to get so low that it's causing fatigue, dizziness, and mental slowing—effects that could be confused with dementia.

TREATMENT FOR HYPERTENSION AND OTHER CARDIOVASCULAR PROBLEMS

When lifestyle changes alone don't result in lower blood pressure or better cardiovascular health, your doctor may recommend drug treatment. Drugs may be aimed at lowering your blood pressure; slowing, stopping, or reversing the buildup of plaque; minimizing the risk of blood clots; treating symptoms; or lowering other risks.

Although nearly all heart medications have side effects that need to be managed, millions have been helped by these life-saving treatments, which have become safer and easier to use in recent years. Statin drugs, for example, have been shown to significantly lower the risk of heart attack and stroke in people who have high blood cholesterol.

And when drug treatment is not enough to reduce your risk of death from heart disease, your doctor may recommend procedures or surgery. Examples include angioplasty, a nonsurgical method for opening blocked or narrowed arteries by inserting a small balloon into the artery and inflating it to compress the plaque against the artery wall so that blood can flow more freely. Patients often receive stents, devices that keep the coronary artery open as part of the angioplasty procedure. Another alternative is bypass surgery, where arteries or veins from other areas of the body are used to bypass, or go around, the area of the coronary artery that's narrowed or blocked.

As with drugs, the development of such procedures has revolutionized the way we think about and treat cardiovascular problems. Millions more people survive heart disease today than they did thirty or forty years ago because of the success of such treatments. Many boomers may recall their parents talking about a relative's heart condition in very grave terms. Millions of boomers lost their own fathers to sudden heart attacks when the men were in their fifties or sixties. That would be much less likely to happen today because of the great progress we've made in preventing and treating heart disease.

But we need to realize that treatments as invasive as bypass surgery, for example, come at a great cost—including the risk of complications and adverse outcomes as patients undergo surgery and recover from it.

That's why it's so much better to proactively avoid the need for such measures, if possible, through healthy lifestyles. And we must also realize how important it is for those with cardiovascular disease who are benefiting from drugs, surgery, and other treatments to make healthy living an integral part of their lives as well. Medical intervention can certainly save the lives of people with serious cardiovascular problems. But good habits like quitting tobacco, exercising regularly, eating a healthy diet, and managing stress are key to experiencing a better life following such intervention.

One of the great joys of practicing internal medicine for so many years is that I have seen many patients adopt extremely healthy lifestyles and treatment plans after cardiac events such as a heart attack or bypass surgery, and live long, active, fulfilling lives.

ABOVE ALL, STOP SMOKING

If you smoke, quitting tobacco is probably the single most effective way to improve your health and build your physical reserves. Smoking harms your body in many ways. It puts you at much higher risk for many cancers and chronic diseases. It damages your blood vessels, which can lead to both high blood pressure and high blood cholesterol—raising your risk of heart attack, stroke, and dementia.

But quitting smoking can improve your health no matter what your age. Within just days of your last cigarette, your body begins to heal from the damage smoking causes. Just one year after you quit, you're half as likely to die of coronary artery disease. After ten years, your risk of dying of lung cancer is cut in half.[10]

Unfortunately, the addictive nature of tobacco use makes it extremely hard for most people to stop. Of all the addictive substances that have been studied, nicotine is the worst. Surprisingly, brain studies show that nicotine is more addictive than heroin, cocaine, or alcohol.

Still, quitting tobacco is not impossible. According to the Centers for Disease Control and Prevention (CDC), more than half of all adult smokers have stopped.[11] Millions who were once addicted to cigarettes are now living smoke free, proving it can be done.

What's the best way to quit? Research shows that combining behavioral counseling with medications—like nicotine patches, bupropion, and varenicline (Chantix)—works best.[12] Counseling is available through hospitals, workplaces, and community groups. Internet- and phone-based support programs staffed by trained counselors have proven to be especially effective because they're so easy to access. These "quit lines," which were first developed at Group Health, are now covered by most health insurance programs. Phone apps and other digital tools are also proving to be a helpful resource for soon-to-be ex-smokers.

Smoking cessation can lead to weight gain, so monitoring your weight while quitting is important. But even if a person gains the typical few pounds, the benefit to blood pressure control and lowered risk of heart attack, stroke, lung cancer, and other illness is more than enough to offset the risk of a modest weight gain.

TAKE IT TO HEART: EXERCISE TRULY *IS* THE BEST MEDICINE

I recently came across an editorial from a 1980s medical journal that I had saved because I thought it was so important. Now, after thirty years, it almost made me laugh. The author asked which is better for heart health: beta-blocker heart drugs or exercise?

First, I was amused by the author's false dichotomy: nobody needs to choose between medicine and exercise. I also found his reasoning odd. He praised the superior effects of physical activity: it was safer and more beneficial. But then he came down on the side of the drug. Why?

Because he believed his patients would never choose the effort of physical activity over the ease of taking a daily pill.

How far we've come in thirty years, I thought. We can now state with unabashed certainty that exercise helps people avoid all kinds of illness: heart attacks, stroke, diabetes, dementia, and so on. Research shows it lowers blood pressure and reduces levels of harmful cholesterol in the blood. It strengthens our bones and muscles. It reduces stress and lifts our moods.

So patients today *gladly* choose exercise; that's why the vast majority of people in Western societies are so healthy and physically fit, right? But of course that's not true. I thought of examples like the landmark 2016 study among a million people published in the *Lancet* that showed less than a quarter were physically active an hour or more a day.[13] And suddenly the old essay didn't seem so amusing anymore. After all these years, and all the scientific research proving the benefits of exercise, the challenge still remains. We must find ways to overcome our inertia. We must find the motivation to become more physically active.

I was reminded of all I learned while working with Robert A. Bruce, the UW cardiologist who pioneered the field of rehabilitation for heart patients. Dr. Bruce first demonstrated that supervised regular exercise was not dangerous but protective for people being treated for cardiovascular illness.[14] But he was also known for discovering that people are not naturally motivated to "just do it" as the Nike ads implore. In research done on his CAPRI program, he found that almost half the people enrolled participated for only six months; at two years, only about 30 percent were still exercising.[15] Despite having suffered a heart attack, the majority were not as motivated to participate in cardiac rehab as one might predict.

And yet I've known many people in my medical practice, research, and professional and social circles who have managed to make daily exercise a regular priority despite legitimate obstacles. Among younger people, motivation often seems to come from wanting to look good or to achieve some recreational goal—climb that mountain or participate in that marathon.

Among people in middle age, I see many motivated by a new diagnosis or health challenge. If it's hypertension or high cholesterol, they see that exercise and a healthy diet may help them avoid the need for a lifelong drug regime, along with its associated side effects. In fact, many of my patients have reduced the number of medications they need for these conditions by upping their physical activity and adopting a better diet.

And sometimes, other illnesses or injuries may be the wake-up call needed to begin an exercise habit. Remember Wayne Grytting, the retired schoolteacher at the end of chapter 2 who was able to avoid—or at least postpone—knee surgery through physical activity and weight loss.

But for many people age sixty or so, I see a more universal incentive come to the fore: people simply want more time on this earth, and they want the energy and well-being it takes to enjoy it. That's why I tell nearly *all* my patients, no matter what their age or condition, that exercise can help them live longer and feel better. And sometimes the message actually gets through.

George Neilson was one of those who took my advice to heart. In his sixties when he first came to my practice, he barely had enough breath to walk down the corridor of my clinic without stopping to rest. His heart was so damaged by atherosclerosis that his cardiologist described his condition as "end-stage" heart disease. He was taking all the appropriate medications for his condition but getting very little physical activity.

George seemed surprised when I suggested that he take short daily walks to improve his stamina. Perhaps he felt fearful, as many heart patients do, that exertion would bring about a heart attack. I assured him that if he took it slowly at first, he would steadily build up his stamina and could exercise without worry. He said he would try it.

George started with very short walks near his house, but within a few months he was taking daily outings of nearly an hour in duration. Eventually, he was even walking in a hilly neighborhood nearby. Sometimes he became breathless, he told me, but that didn't keep him home. He would simply stop, catch his breath, and then move on.

George continued this routine for many years—more than I ever expected him to live. What difference did it make? He did not experience the level of decline people with end-stage heart disease usually have. I believe that's because his daily walks kept his skeletal muscles toned, which placed lower demands on his heart muscle. The exercise also helped him keep a positive attitude. He was happy to get out of his house every day, see neighbors, and enjoy the great outdoors.

BUT HOW MUCH EXERCISE IS ENOUGH?

For the health of your heart and blood vessels, the answer is fairly simple: your goal should be at least thirty to sixty minutes a day—every day. And more is generally better.

But if you're new to exercise and an hour of daily physical activity feels like too much, don't be discouraged. Just start slowly and work up to it. Our research shows that even small amounts of exercise are better than none at all. In one study of our ACT seniors aged sixty-five and older, for example, we found that people who exercised more than fifteen minutes three days a week had a 30 to 40 percent lower risk of Alzheimer's disease and dementia than those who exercised less.[16] The bottom line: Shun the couch-potato existence. Get up and exercise even if only for a short time. Avoid being sedentary.

Strive to make some of your exercise time aerobic, which means that your heart beats somewhat faster than usual and you're breathing a little harder. Some experts recommend that at least ten minutes of each exercise session be aerobic. But again, more is probably better.

The most important thing is to make exercise *a habit*—like brushing your teeth or feeding the dog. It's something you do every day; you wouldn't think of *not* doing it. And some people find it helpful to schedule physical activity at the same time every day—say, right after breakfast or before dinner. This minimizes uncertainty about if and when you're going to do it.

Another key is to choose forms of exercise you really enjoy. If exercise feels like drudgery, you may be setting yourself up for failure. So think about activities that really appeal to you—whether that's walking in nature, swimming laps in a pool, joining a gym or exercise class, or using a fitness machine in the privacy of your own home.

Brisk walking is probably the easiest. You can do it nearly anywhere, and you don't need special skills or equipment—just a pair of comfortable shoes. Weather need not be a deterrent if you can dress for it. But if you find it's too hot, too cold, too wet, or too dark outside, try walking in a shopping mall. Some malls open early just to attract recreational walkers who appreciate the safety of a well-lit, secure environment.

If it's hard for you to find time to exercise, consider combining it with other fun or must-do activities. Read the newspaper while riding a stationary bike. Listen to an audiobook while walking on a treadmill.

Lift hand weights and do squats while watching the TV. Commute to work while riding your bike. Catch up with your best friend while walking outdoors. Actively quiet your mind or pray while swimming in the pool.

GET UP, STAND UP!

You can also boost your physical activity by finding ways to decrease the time you spend in sedentary positions—that is, sitting or lying down. Health scientists have linked such behavior to increased risks of heart disease, diabetes, and some cancers.[17] Now they're exploring the health benefits of coaching people to spend more time on their feet, which might include increased circulation for heart health, stronger bones and muscles, and better weight management due to more calories burned.

Finding ways to sit less can be challenging for those who need to work at a computer eight hours a day. One solution is to raise your workstation to counter height so you can type while standing, a practice that's increasingly common among my colleagues at Group Health Research Institute. (You'll also need a tall chair so you can sit once in a while when fatigue sets in.) Also, you might try standing and stretching occasionally during meetings or when watching television or videos.

If you ride public transportation, you might follow Gerald Alexander's lead. At age eighty-two, Gerald participated in a research study my colleague Dori Rosenberg conducted to encourage seniors to sit less. He often boarded a city bus near his neighborhood high school. Rather than taking a seat, he would grab the handrail and remain standing. "When kids see an old guy standing, they feel like they've got to get up and offer him a seat—and sometimes they'd be quite insistent," he laughed. "I had to really persuade them that, 'No, I enjoy standing.'"[18]

Through their coaching, Dr. Rosenberg's team found that study participants reduced their sitting from an average of eight hours a day to seven and a half. The seniors also started walking faster and reported feeling less depressed and better able to accomplish everyday tasks.[19]

What if there's just no way to avoid hours on your bottom? (Example: You're a full-time bus driver.) The 2016 *Lancet* study I mentioned earlier provided encouraging news.[20] It showed that just one hour per day of physical activity such as brisk walking or cycling could offset the risk of early death from full-time sitting by 12 to 59 percent. The more the participants exercised, the greater protection they got.

But isn't an hour a lot? In my advice to patients, I have typically recommended thirty rather than sixty minutes of exercise per day—especially to people who may not have exercised regularly before.

But I did appreciate what Ulf Ekelund, author of the *Lancet* study, told the press when asked the same question. Daily TV viewing time among adults in the UK is three hours. "Is it too much to ask that just a little of that be devoted to physical activity?" he asked.[21]

Here in the United States, adults spend an average of *four* hours a day watching television. So I think here and probably elsewhere around the world, Dr. Ekelund's point is well taken.

Once you commit to being more physically active, you see opportunities throughout your day: You decide to take the stairs instead of the elevator. You get off the bus a stop or two early and walk the rest of the way. You park at the back of the lot instead of near the door. And you take the grandkids to the park on the way home from the matinee.

As with any effort at behavior change, tracking your progress can inspire success. You can do this simply by writing down the number of minutes you spend each day in various categories of activity—lying down, sitting, exercising, and so on. You can also wear a device that tracks movement for you. A simple mechanical pedometer can count your steps. Or you can use a digital activity tracker, such as a Fitbit, which you can wear on your wrist, at your waist, or in your pocket to monitor a variety of "personal metrics." As with smartphone apps that perform the same function, you can use these activity trackers to monitor calories burned, floors climbed, and duration and intensity of your activity.

Such gizmos can be fun and motivating for some, especially if you're fascinated by data and technology. But remember: you don't need any of this to achieve better fitness. All you need to do is get moving and step up the duration and pace of your activities little by little over time.

It really matters that you pay attention minute by minute to the choices you're making throughout the day. For example, you find yourself feeling restless and realize that you haven't moved from the same spot for hours. So you get up and take a ten-minute stretch and walk.

Such awareness is part of the concept psychologists refer to as "mindfulness," and you can apply it to many aspects of healthy living—

from physical activity to the foods you eat to the way you react emotionally when things get stressful. Being mindful means staying awake to new possibilities rather than operating on "automatic pilot." You surprise yourself throughout your day by saying things like, "I'll walk to the corner market instead of driving to the big store." Or, "I think I'll skip the ice cream and go for nonfat frozen yogurt instead." Or, "I could get really angry at that guy's driving, but it's better for my blood pressure if I just let it go."

HEALTHY DIET MATTERS—FOR YOUR HEART AND OVERALL HEALTH

Perhaps nowhere is mindfulness needed more than at the dining table. Diet plays an essential role in controlling your risk for cardiovascular disease and building other physical reserves. Along with regular exercise, eating well can help you to keep your blood pressure and blood cholesterol in check and to manage your weight—all of which is important for protecting your heart and blood vessels as well as many other body parts.

But what constitutes a healthy diet? I believe the best advice is fairly simple:

- Eat more fruits and vegetables.
- Use nonfat or low-fat dairy foods.
- Cut back on foods high in saturated fat, cholesterol, and trans fat.
- Eat more whole-grain foods, fish, poultry, and nuts.
- Limit sodium, sweets, sugary drinks, and red meats.

These guidelines come from the DASH diet, which stands for "Dietary Approaches to Stop Hypertension." (But if that doesn't sound very appealing to you, call it the "Mediterranean diet," which takes a similar approach.)

DASH was designed by the National Heart, Lung, and Blood Institute (NHLBI) for people with high blood pressure and high blood cholesterol, and it's good for just about everybody else as well. You can go to the NHLBI website for more details about how it works.[22]

But once you commit to a heart-healthy diet, you'll find yourself steering clear of many popular fast-food restaurants, which tend to push foods high in salt, sugar, and saturated fats. (This includes foods with a high glycemic index, the kind of carbohydrates that cause spikes in blood sugar and make you want to eat more—very good for profits, but not for health.) You can still eat out; just look for places that focus on fresh fruits and vegetables instead of highly processed and packaged foods.

Generally, however, cooking at home has advantages. You can better control how much salt and sodium you're getting, for example. Low-salt food doesn't have to be dull if you add more herbs and spices. If you have high blood pressure, talk to your doctor or dietician about how much you should limit sodium in your diet.

I've learned a lot about healthy home cooking from my wife, Teresa Bigelow, whose mom had high blood pressure. Her family never ate fast food, and she never acquired a taste for salt. We build our meals around fruits and vegetables, with modest servings of animal protein and starch. We always have a fresh salad with tasty dressings based on olive oil, herbs, and tangy lemon or vinegars, usually at the end of the main plate and before taking an extra helping. We don't use creamy dressings. She even seasons cooked green vegetables with lemon, not the butter I grew up eating.

You'll want to be discerning about the fats and oils you use. Saturated fats are those that are hard at room temperature: butter, lard, meat fat, solid shortening, palm oil, and coconut oil. And you'll also want to limit foods made with hydrogenated oils and fats, such as stick margarine, and baked goods, such as cookies, cakes and pies, crackers, frostings, and coffee creamers.

Not all fats are bad, however. Monounsaturated and polyunsaturated fats actually help lower blood cholesterol levels. Sources include avocados; olive, corn, canola, and soybean oils; nuts and seeds; salmon and trout; and tofu. But you can't eat unlimited amounts of these foods because most are also high in calories.

And finally, it's best to limit alcohol. Too much alcohol raises your blood pressure and triglyceride levels, a type of fat found in the blood. It also adds calories, causing weight gain. Guidelines call for men to have no more than two drinks a day; women, no more than one drink a day. One drink is twelve ounces of beer, five ounces of wine, or one and a half ounces of liquor. (Yes, these guidelines may seem restrictive, especially for "social drinkers" who enjoy more alcohol on special occasions. But please remember: alcohol puts people at risk for falls. Tragically, I've seen many older people suffer serious concussions or fractures from falling—often down stairs—after "just a couple drinks" at celebratory dinners or parties. My advice: if you drink, always do so in moderation.)

AN EVERYDAY COMMITMENT TO HEALTHY WEIGHT

If you're overweight, a healthy diet and exercise can go a long way toward losing pounds for better health—and proactively building physical reserves for old age. Losing weight may lower your risk for high blood pressure, high cholesterol, diabetes, joint pain, cancer, and many other problems. If you've already been diagnosed with an obesity-related chronic illness, weight loss may help to alleviate many problems. And in some cases, it can help you avoid harmful medications and invasive procedures and surgeries.

Despite these benefits, however, weight management is difficult for many. In fact, of all the health challenges the boomer generation faces, our society's obesity epidemic may be the most daunting. Public health officials now estimate that about two-thirds of American adults are either overweight or obese. Most experts define overweight as having a body mass index—or BMI—of 25 or greater; obesity is a BMI of 30 or more. Although there is some emerging evidence that for seniors, a BMI between 25 and 30 may not be as risky as previously thought, if your BMI is 30 or above, your health risks are certainly increased. And more Americans than ever before are now in this range.

How did this happen to our population? The problem is linked to widespread social changes over a period of decades. Throughout Western society, people are spending increasingly more time sitting still to watch television or to work and play at computers. Also, with more dual-income households, families are cooking at home less and relying more on high-calorie take-out and processed foods. Meanwhile, the availability of calorie-dense convenience foods has increased dramatically. Hard-to-resist junk food is available everywhere—office buildings, schools, hospitals, shopping malls, hardware stores—you name it.

One study showed that, excluding the kind of stores that typically sell food (i.e., groceries stores, convenience stores, liquor stores, and restaurants), 41 percent of commercial establishments display or sell foods to their patrons. It wasn't always like this. The snack and fast-food industries have honed their marketing to take advantage of our attraction to sugar and fat. At the same time, it's gotten harder for many people—especially those in low-income neighborhoods—to get access to affordable healthy foods like fresh fruits and vegetables. Convenience foods yield a higher profit.

Understanding the social causes of our obesity epidemic can be useful on many levels. It can help communities to develop public health–oriented solutions. It may also help us to stop blaming weight problems on individuals' lack of "will power." This, in turn, may help overweight people to seek the support they need to change their eating patterns and physical activity over the long haul.

And make no mistake: changing eating behavior is not easy. Scientists have discovered how high-fat, high-sugar foods tend to trigger the release of the feel-good chemical dopamine in pleasure centers of the brain, so that we're not only attracted to such foods in the first place; we're also driven to keep going back for more.[23] This trait may have helped our species survive starvation thousands of years ago. But now that our environment is saturated with high-calorie food, the setup is literally killing us.

How then can overweight individuals develop the motivation to resist such pressures? It's a tough question, and aimed at a key element for improving health: the individual's enduring commitment to make choices moment by moment that will help them feel better over the long haul. Unfortunately, research shows that the majority of overweight people who lose a substantial number of pounds give up the struggle eventually and return to their original weight.

But does it really have to be this way? Again, this is where my optimism about boomers gets triggered. What if we could harness our generation's interest in self-actualization and activism to truly change the game when it comes to eating and exercise? We have learned so much in recent years—through science and from our friends and families—about the way lifestyle changes can improve health for people as we age. We also know that many of us are expected to live into our nineties and beyond, and we want to be well enough to enjoy those years. Weight management is difficult, but what if knowledge about healthy aging could bring unprecedented motivation to the issue? I'm hopeful that by sharing ideas about enlightened aging, we'll be able to inspire more individuals than ever before to make everyday commitments to those behaviors that can sustain a healthy weight—resulting in a happier, healthier life in old age.

A FEW BASICS ABOUT WEIGHT LOSS

I encourage my patients who are overweight to set targets to monitor their progress regularly. By consistently losing two to three pounds a month, you can lose between twenty-five and thirty pounds in a year. That can make a significant difference in helping people with hypertension to lower their blood pressure. It may also address other problems, such as lowering blood cholesterol, decreasing your risk of diabetes, and alleviating knee or hip pain.

Weight loss programs can be helpful. I've seen people succeed with supervised programs, such as Weight Watchers, which provides solid teaching and peer support. I've seen others avoid the cost of such programs by designing their own, using guidelines like the DASH diet, supplemented with online resources or calorie-counting phone apps. And I've seen people do well by enrolling in expensive programs that provide meals, exercise classes, and individualized behavioral counseling.

Whichever way you go, if you commit to several months of steady, active participation, you have a good chance of losing weight the way that's best for health—that is, gradually, a few pounds per month. So-called crash diets are not good for you. Indeed, they produce a pattern of yo-yo weight gains and losses that are particularly bad for health and long-term weight control.

So be an enlightened activist. Find a plan that makes sense for you and stick with it. Don't think of your effort as "a diet" or a campaign that you're going to try for a few months and then drop. That attitude will just get you back where you started. Focus instead on the changes you're making day by day to live a longer, healthier life.

And what if you find that you're eating well and exercising but not losing weight? You might talk to your doctor, a dietician, or a weight-loss counselor for advice. But don't get discouraged: even people who, according to their BMI, are overweight can gain added protection against heart disease and stroke by having a regular exercise program and lowering their blood pressure. Research has shown that it's better to be "fit and fat" than it is to be out of shape and at a normal weight. Remember: keep moving and your health will benefit!

LETTING GO OF STRESS—FOR HEART HEALTH AND MORE

Research shows that reducing stress can also help some people control their blood pressure, reducing their risk for cardiovascular disease and other illnesses. In addition, finding ways to relax and let go of anxiety may improve the quality of our lives in general.

I often have an opportunity to teach patients with stress-related hypertension about relaxation during a routine physical exam. I start by taking the patient's blood pressure once or twice to get a baseline. Then I ask them to close their eyes and take several breaths—in and out, slowly and deeply, through slightly pursed lips, which slows the airflow. After about ten breaths, I take the patient's blood pressure again. Many experience a drop of 10 to 30 millimeters of mercury (mmHg). Although basic, the exercise immediately demonstrates the power some individuals may have to significantly affect their own blood pressure—simply by taking a few minutes of slow, measured breathing to relax.

Much of Western medicine's interest in stress reduction for health began with research by Harvard cardiologist Herbert Benson. He founded the Institute for Mind Body Medicine after writing *The Relaxation Response* in 1975.[24] His book describes how meditation can reduce the body's production of the hormones epinephrine and norepinephrine (aka adrenaline), which causes our blood pressure to spike when we're under high stress. This "fight or flight" physiological response may have helped our prehistoric ancestors escape danger. It raises our blood pressure, increases our heart rate and breathing, and dilates our pupils, for example—all helpful responses when fleeing a tiger. Only nowadays, stress is more likely to come from problems like family quarrels, pressure at work, or an ugly commute—that is, challenges from which we don't typically flee. But we still experience the physiological stress of the fight-or-flight response, which can lead to chronic health problems like hypertension, chest pain, tension headaches, back pain, and so on.

But Dr. Benson and many others since have observed that when people learn to respond to stress in a more relaxed way, they can experience healthy decreases in blood pressure, heart rate, and muscle tension. That "relaxation response" can be taught through various forms of meditation, yoga, prayer, biofeedback, and breathing and muscle relaxation techniques.

As one of my early med school mentors, Dr. Benson and his work made a big impression on me. It's highly relevant for older people especially—as high blood pressure becomes increasingly more common with age. By age ninety, most people will be diagnosed with hypertension. To help my patients avoid associated cardiovascular problems, I almost always recommend each person find and practice a way to actively relax their body and state of mind. This can involve learning new behaviors you've never tried before—say, meditation, quiet prayer, chanting, or consciously taking deep, soothing breaths when you're under stress. Or it may be something that you've been doing your whole life, and just practicing it more consistently.

Relaxation practices such as calming prayer or meditation can help people manage stressful thoughts that cause emotional upset and fight-or-flight responses. Meditation has been proven to be helpful for a variety of stress-related problems, including hypertension, anxiety, and chronic pain.[25] One example is a form of meditation called mindfulness-based stress reduction, which is becoming increasingly popular in the United States. This technique involves training in observing, acknowledging, and accepting thoughts and feelings in the moment. It can also include some easy yoga poses, which help people become more immediately aware of their bodies—including their breath and muscle tension.

Whether today's enlightened agers will be more open to simple, commonsense approaches to controlling stress than previous generations is unknown. The growing popularity of yoga, meditation, and other forms of group and individual stress-reduction practices is a hopeful trend. A 2012 survey from the National Center for Complementary and Integrative Health showed that nearly 10 percent of U.S. adults practiced yoga that year, up from 5 percent a decade earlier.[26] Presumably this includes those who participate in "gentle yoga" or "senior yoga" classes, which are becoming increasingly popular in senior communities and elsewhere.

Another hopeful observation is that people seem to experience less chronic daily stress as they age. Illness, the death of loved ones, relocation, and loss of independence can create periods of debilitating upset for seniors. But as I described in chapter 1, research shows that older people's life experiences commonly provide them with the wisdom and equanimity to weather such changes.

I have also observed how prayer and worship can serve as a great consolation for people as they age. My boomer friends have sometimes commented that most people regularly attending services in mainstream denominations are so old. I figure that's happening for good reason: the elderly, more than others, recognize the value of such practice.

I remember one patient in particular—a retired physician who was nearing the end of her life and feeling quite anxious about her decline. But as time passed, I noticed that something shifted. Her demeanor seemed more and more serene, and I wasn't sure why. Then, shortly before her death, I learned that she had started attending Mass every day. Although she had always been a devout Roman Catholic, she had not worshipped with such frequency until those last stages of her life. By actively practicing her faith on a daily basis near the end, she felt more peaceful.

Many people also find physical activity—especially aerobic exercise—helpful for controlling stress and anxiety. This is likely related to the same reasons that exercise contributes to the overall health of the brain, which we discussed at length in chapter 5. It increases blood flow to the brain, delivering the building blocks of oxygen, nutrients, and other materials that the brain needs in order to function well. This includes the delivery of endorphins, the hormone that produces "runner's high"—the euphoria that athletes sometimes feel following long, intense periods of physical exertion. But you don't have to be a marathon runner to experience an improved mood from exercising. People just naturally tend to feel better emotionally after moving about. It's part of the human condition, and I encourage you to experiment with it when you're under stress.

And don't forget that counseling may also help you to manage stress—particularly if you're looking for new perspectives for enduring problems around job pressures, relationship problems, or other life circumstances. Many people find that cognitive behavioral therapy is particularly good for such difficulties because it focuses on helping you "reframe" your thoughts, beliefs, and attitudes about your troubles. The idea is that changing the way you think can change the way you feel. Also, unlike many forms of psychotherapy, and especially psychoanalysis, Cognitive behavioral therapy is generally time limited; clients learn skills they can use on their own to handle stressful situations. Counseling may also provide tools to help you talk through conflicts with family members, friends, or coworkers. Ideally, you'll be less stressed, which is better for your overall health and well-being.

MAINTAIN HEARING FOR RESILIENCE

While most people experience some age-related hearing loss over time, activated seniors resist passively attributing such changes to "just getting old." Instead, they consider ways to prevent further losses, maintain the function they still have, and adapt to limitations they're experiencing.

Hearing loss affects about one in three people in the United States between ages sixty-five and seventy-four. By age seventy-five, half of all people have trouble hearing.[27] Just because it's common, however, doesn't make it easy to live with. Depending on severity, hearing loss can cause stress in relationships because of miscommunication. It can be a safety concern if you're having difficulty hearing certain kinds of instructions, alarms, or announcements. Trouble participating in conversations, hearing the television, or listening to the speaker at an important event can leave you feeling socially isolated.

Hearing problems can result from health conditions such as high blood pressure or diabetes. Exposure to noise that's too loud or lasts too long can also cause hearing loss. (Note that a study of older people who had lived their entire lives in the quiet of Easter Island showed they had far better hearing than their counterparts who had moved to industrialized areas.) So if you've worked around loud machinery, firearms, sirens, loud music, or so on, you may be at risk.[28]

You can minimize further damage by avoiding unnecessary clatter. Don't use headsets or ear buds at loud volume, for example. And wear earplugs if you're still being exposed to loud noise on a regular basis.

Typically, hearing problems develop over time, and you may not notice how bad your loss has become until you've had a series of stressful or annoying incidents where you wished things had gone differently. Maybe it was a meeting or family event where you felt left out because you couldn't hear over background noise or you thought somebody was speaking too softly. Then suddenly it dawns on you that the problem isn't them; it's your hearing.

Once you decide to get your hearing assessed, talk to your doctor. You'll probably be referred to an audiologist, who will test your hearing and may suggest you get a hearing aid. In case you haven't noticed, today's hearing aids are typically much smaller and less obtrusive than they were decades ago. And new technology has also made them much easier to use. But if you get one and find you're having trouble adjusting to it, be persistent in asking questions about how to make it work for you. Most people I know who have hearing aids tell me that it took some getting used to, but eventually they were glad they made the effort because hearing well again has improved their lives. And don't put it off because the longer you wait, the more you'll miss.

In addition, you may want to try using assisted listening devices (ALDs), which are often available to people with hearing loss when they attend large facilities such as classrooms, theaters, or places of worship. Some organizations also have them available for use in small settings for one-on-one conversations. ALDs can amplify sounds you want to hear without picking up background noises. They can be used independently or in concert with a hearing aid.

One more thought: Many people learn to enhance their hearing by supplementing what they hear with what they see. In other words, they learn to "read lips," a skill that grows easier with practice. I have been surprised at how many of my patients do this successfully. Here are two tips I've learned from them: (1) Always place yourself where you can see the speaker's face. (2) Tell friends and relatives that you're doing this so they can cooperate.

Most importantly, resist the urge to withdraw because of hearing problems. Dropping out of social interactions hastens age-related decline, so keep communicating!

PROTECT YOUR VISION TOO

It also pays to take an active stance toward maintaining your eyesight and adjusting to changes as they occur. Two key factors to maintaining healthy eyesight are the following:

1. *Regular, comprehensive dilated eye exams:* Such exams will help you keep prescription eyeglasses up-to-date. But more importantly, they are the only way to detect certain eye diseases that can lead to severe vision problems if left untreated. These include glaucoma, diabetic retinopathy, and age-related macular degeneration.

2. *A healthy lifestyle:* Diabetes is a risk factor for diabetic retinopathy, glaucoma, and cataracts. So manage your weight and exercise regularly to prevent diabetes from developing. Smoking puts you at higher risk for macular degeneration and cataracts, so don't smoke. Also, eat a diet rich in fruits and vegetables (especially dark leafy greens) and fish high in omega-3 fatty acids such as salmon, tuna, and halibut. These foods have been linked to a lower risk for certain eye diseases.

Age-related macular degeneration is the leading cause of severe visual impairment among people sixty and older. It happens when the macula, a small center portion of the retina, which is located at the back of the eye, deteriorates. Macular degeneration doesn't cause complete blindness, but it blurs images in the center of your vision, interfering with "straight-ahead" activities such as reading, driving, and recognizing faces. Treatments, which can slow the progression of the disease, include medicine injected into the eye or laser therapy.

Diabetic retinopathy, the most common type of diabetes-related eye disease, is a risk for people with both type 1 and type 2 diabetes. The longer you have diabetes, the greater your risk. Retinopathy changes the blood vessels in the back part of the eye, the retina, causing them to bleed or leak fluid and distort vision. Left untreated, it can cause severe vision loss and blindness. People with diabetes can prevent diabetic retinopathy by taking their medications as prescribed, staying physically active, and maintaining a healthy diet. Treatments such as eyedrops and eye injections are available if retinopathy occurs, and carefully adhering to them can prevent more severe vision loss.

Glaucoma is a group of diseases that damage the optic nerve, interfering at first with peripheral (side) vision. Over time, glaucoma also affects straight-ahead vision and, left untreated, can eventually lead to blindness. Glaucoma can be treated with medicine, surgery, or other procedures. These treatments can save remaining vision, but they can't restore vision that's already been lost. That's why it's so important to catch the disease early. Anyone can get glaucoma, but it tends to run in families. The risk is higher for African Americans over age forty and anyone over age sixty, especially Mexican Americans.

Cataracts are cloudy tissues on the lens of your eye that can block light from entering the retina and make your vision blurry. Certain diseases, such as diabetes, put you at higher risk. So do smoking, alcohol use, and prolonged exposure to sunlight. The most common treatment is outpatient surgery. Fortunately, I see increasingly more people choosing this treatment. As with hearing aids, successful cataract surgery can dramatically improve older people's ability to stay actively engaged in their lives.

And what happens when, despite preventive measures and treatments, visual impairment can't be corrected with surgery, eyeglasses, or medicines? Many older people still take steps to prevent vision problems from interfering with their everyday activities.

I'm reminded of seniors like Evangeline Shuler, who switched to audiobooks when she could no longer read the biographies she enjoyed. I also think of Lena Feldman, the ninety-three-year-old wife of an ACT study participant I mentioned in chapter 1. When her vision problems made it difficult to read the newspaper, she switched to an online version of the *New York Times*. Her computer allows her to make the font as large as she needs. And because she can no longer drive, she's using her computer to order groceries online and schedule shuttle rides to the doctor.

These are just a few simple examples of the ways new devices can make life easier for people with visual impairments.

If you have vision problems that interfere with your everyday activities, ask your doctor about organizations in your community that help people with impaired vision. Many universities and community organizations offer services such as training to use assistive devices, help with home modifications (such as improved lighting), and assistance for developing strategies to navigate inside and outside the home.

Remember: as age-related changes come your way, it pays to think in terms of building and maintaining your reserves. For functions like vision and hearing, this means recognizing and adapting to problems when they occur. Doing so can help you stay as physically and socially active as possible.

In the next chapter, we'll learn more about building your social reserves, which is another important aspect of staying strong and resilient as time goes by.

7

BUILDING YOUR SOCIAL RESERVES

Just as we need to build our mental and physical reserves for resilience in old age, we need to build our social reserves—that is, the network of people and resources that allows us to have a safe, comfortable, stable place to grow old.

Simply put, it's much better to grow old when you're surrounded by friends and relatives who care about your health, your safety, and your well-being. Most of the benefits are pretty obvious—especially as we face age-related changes such as limited mobility or the loss of loved ones. Lending a hand to each other in illness, grief, and disability is what friends and family do. But other perks of living and working in a strong community may not be so apparent. For example, avoiding social isolation makes us more resilient; we're better able to bounce back from illness when it happens.

How social reserves come together for any individual depends on a wide range of factors, such as your culture, your family situation, and your finances. There are many questions to consider: Where will you live? How long will you continue working? How will you spend your leisure time? How much money will you need to have saved? Who will be your helpers and your advocates when needed?

These are very personal questions that only you and your family can answer. What's most important is to be proactive and begin planning early so the resources will be in place when you need them.

While it can be hard to predict what you'll need or want in the future, research on seniors' preferences points to common concerns.

For example, when my colleagues and I asked our ACT study participants about their perceptions of successful aging, we learned that having a sense of autonomy was important to most as they grew older. At the same time, they want to stay involved with others. They don't want to feel isolated or lonely. They want to keep learning. And they certainly don't want to feel that they're a burden to others. All of these issues can be influenced by where people live, who surrounds them, and whom they can rely on.

Obviously, creating a strong social network for ourselves does not happen overnight. Also, it's impossible to know who among our family and friends will still be there for us as we grow old. Indeed, we don't really know how much help we're going to need or when. Dependency is something nobody wants, and it may be hard to admit that it can happen to you. But if we live long enough, chances are high that we'll need at least some assistance—whether from our friends, relatives, or professional helpers and caregivers.

Early on, you may not require much help—maybe a hand with housecleaning, yard work, or home repairs. But later, your needs may grow to include help with driving, paying bills, getting meals, and so on. And eventually, as you face challenges with memory and mobility, you're likely to need a lot more assistance with many functions of everyday life.

If thinking about a future where you must rely on others makes you uncomfortable, you're not alone. I believe it's human nature to hope that we can stay independent as long as possible. And indeed, the "compression of morbidity" I described in chapter 4 may allow many to postpone disability until very late in life. That means it's likely we'll need help for at least some period. According to the National Institute on Aging, about 70 percent of people over age sixty-five will need some type of long-term care during their lifetime. More than 40 percent need care in a nursing home for some period.[1] To deny that we'll need such extra help as we age is like trying to deny hair loss or wrinkles. We can buy a toupee or skin cream, but these things are still going to occur.

That's why it's best to (1) accept that changes are likely to come with age, and (2) take steps now to preserve and enhance your social and financial reserves. By doing so, you'll be in the best possible position to enjoy your later years.

WHY ELDER CARE IS DIFFERENT TODAY

Generations ago, it was typically assumed that a younger (and usually female) relative—say, a daughter or daughter-in-law—would provide elder care within families. But societal changes over the past several decades have made such assumptions obsolete for many Americans. With more women in the workplace, fewer are home to look after elderly relatives. Also, families are smaller, and more people are choosing not to have kids at all. Therefore, the number of relatives available to share the responsibility of caring for elderly family members is shrinking.

At the same time, longer life expectancy means the caregiver's job lasts longer. The financial burden can also be greater, especially if an elderly family member survives longer than their retirement plan ever anticipated.

Also, with longer life spans, some families are juggling the needs of two generations of elderly—say, grandma in her seventies and great-grandma in her nineties. In addition, divorce and remarriage gives some families more than their standard share of elderly dependents; in addition to two sets of grandparents, for example, they've got granddad's second wife and grandma's common-law husband. And that doesn't even include older aunts or uncles who are childless and may look to extended family for assistance.

The transient nature of our society also adds to the load. Families used to stick together in one community for generations. But now it's more common for relatives to spread out geographically, leaving fewer folks to take responsibility for mom and dad's care. In cases where nobody's nearby, adult children struggle to arrange for an elder parents' care from afar.

Adventurous aged retirees don't make it any easier on their grown children. I remember how worried my sister and I became when my parents were in their eighties and still spending winters in a remote area of Arizona. Ever since they had retired and bought a trailer there, Dad liked to meander in the desert, stopping to chat with his few neighbors and enjoy the outdoors. Likewise, Mom loved the cacti, sunsets, and warm weather—a contrast to wet, cold Oregon winters. But as they grew older and began to slow down, my sister and I became increasingly nervous. How could we ensure their well-being when we could not even reach them by phone? Eventually, they left the trailer for a condo in a town nearby where a cousin lived. But even then, the distance was worrisome to us. Looking back, I'm glad they had those happy years living independently before they grew too frail. But I was also relieved when they later decided to move back to the Pacific Northwest.

I think it's safe to say that most families want to do all they can to keep their elderly loved ones safe and well cared for. And doing so may come more easily for some families than for others. That seemed to be the case for my patient Rolando Perez, who died at age ninety-nine in the home he shared with his daughter. Rolando's vitality in old age was really quite remarkable. If you ask his daughters, they credit his strong, close-knit web of friends and relatives—a safety net he had a large part in creating.

"WHATEVER YOU GIVE, YOU WILL GET BACK"

In his late nineties, Rolando still recognized his five children, nine grandchildren, fifteen great-grandchildren, and two great-great-grand-children who gathered for his birthday parties. Remembering each of their names, however, was a different matter.

"I know you!" he would say, pointing at each with a mischievous grin. "You are . . . the child of your mother!" Then, chuckling, he would invite the little ones to join him in a round of dominoes.

That's how Rolando handled most challenges of aging—with good humor and grace. Even as he struggled with his failing memory, eyesight, and hearing, he rarely seemed discouraged. "He was just a very happy person," said his daughter Barbara Perez.[2]

Rolando came to the United States from the Philippines with his wife, Maria, and two of their five daughters in 1968—a year after their son was recruited to work for Boeing in Seattle. Sadly, Maria died of lung cancer less than a year after they arrived. Rolando turned his focus to raising his girls and earning enough to send them and other relatives to college. Trained as a teacher in the Philippines, Rolando also had a law degree. Here in the United States, he found a job translating technical manuals.

After retirement, Rolando constantly found enterprising ways to stay active in Seattle's Filipino American community. He became a notary public and helped his clients draw up wills, prepare taxes, or deal with issues related to immigration or divorce. He helped friends and family with term papers, job applications, and résumés. He had a service videotaping weddings and parties. For fun, he liked going to nightclubs and casinos, line dancing, playing the saxophone and clarinet, and entertaining the kids with magic tricks.

Rolando stayed active physically and socially well into his nineties. Each day, he walked eight blocks to the grocery store for lottery tickets. On Sundays, he walked to Mass.

When Barbara's work as a research manager required her to travel from time to time, she would hire a professional caregiver to stay with him at night. She wanted to be sure he got his medications and evening meals. But otherwise, she felt he was safe at home with friends and relatives dropping by.

"I don't think he got lonely at all," his daughter Rebecca Perez, a pediatrician, added. "He had a big family that came to visit him a lot."[3]

"Plus, for all his birthdays, we would have a family get-together," said Barbara. As years passed, the parties grew more elaborate. Once it was a cruise to Mexico. Another time, they gathered in Las Vegas. And one year, they rented a big house on Washington's Olympic Peninsula. "He loved the get-togethers and he loved the attention!" she added.

Was Rolando happy because of his close family ties, or did the relatives stay close to him because of his good nature? I suspect it worked both ways. Also, Rolando's Filipino culture—which places a high value on family connections—encouraged the Perez's interdependency.

"Somehow, most American families believe the farther away you get from your parents the better," said Rebecca. But she and her sister feel just the opposite. "When the parents get older, it's better for somebody in the extended family to take care of them."

The sisters say they remember the sacrifices their dad made for them and other relatives. "If you take care of your family, they will take care of you," said Barbara.

"Whatever you give, you will get back," Rebecca added.

This model of reciprocity seemed to work well for Rolando and his large, close-knit family. But what about the next generation? Neither Barbara nor Rebecca has her own children. Reflecting on this, Barbara could only laugh ironically. "I don't know who is going to take of us," she said with a sigh.

Like many others their age, the Perez sisters may need to look beyond traditional ideas of family-provided care for a different solution. As they do, I urge them to be proactive, considering what matters most based on personal values.

MANY CHOICES—AT A WIDE RANGE OF COSTS

Once you start planning for postretirement housing, care, and finances, you realize there are many options, ranging from various kinds of retirement homes to "aging in place"—that is, staying put in your own home while arranging for help to come to you as needs arise. Understanding the cost and benefits of different arrangements may influence other important decisions, such as how long you want to keep working and how important it is for you to stay near your current community.

While most people place a high value on staying in their own homes as they age, it's important to avoid becoming socially isolated. If people spend too much time alone in old age, they can quickly lose their mental sharpness. It's crucial to be around other people, whether that's with friends and relatives in our own homes, or with other residents of a shared-living situation, such as a retirement community.

Those who have helped their own relatives navigate this complex terrain often have clear notions of what they're after. One example is Ben Stevenson's daughter Linda Tabor, who is seventy-eight. As you may recall from chapter 4, Ben lived independently until a year or so following his accident with his horse. After that, he moved out of state to live with his elderly sister for a few years, followed by stays at two different nursing homes. Linda now realizes that Ben's stay with his sister was isolating for him and may have hastened his decline. Also, the stress of these moves was hard on him mentally and physically—a phenomenon I've observed in other patients as well. Very elderly people generally do better when they can stay in one safe, comfortable environment over time.

So Linda is thinking the best solution for her and her husband would be a retirement community that offers "step" or "progressive" care. That is, residents start out living independently in their own apartments, gradually getting more assistance as needed. Eventually, they may move into the community's nursing facility for specialized care.

(This is the kind of arrangement my parents had during their last years. Like many older people, they initially resisted leaving their home. But once they became accustomed to the "life care" community, the arrangement worked out well for them.)

But Linda hopes that, first, she and her husband can stay in their own home for several more years. To increase their chances of remaining independent for a long time, the couple tries to stay as physically active and healthy as possible. They've also outfitted their bathroom with handrails to prevent falls—often a first step in making a house safer for seniors. (Hearing this I think of ACT study participant Joe Feldman, whom I introduced in chapter 1. At age 101, he's still living independently with his wife Lena, and they are so very careful to avoid falls. For them and for many frail elderly people, fall prevention is part of retaining their social structure. Remember, Joe said, "One bad fall and we know we're out of business."[4] At their age, if either one goes down, they both do.)

Determining the financial costs of various long-term care solutions can be particularly complex. Unless you've arranged care for an elderly relative or friend, you could suffer a bit of "sticker shock" when you see how much it costs to live in various care facilities or to hire caregivers to work in your home. That's why I advise my patients and friends to think about these issues well in advance. While it may be difficult to predict what kind of care you and your loved ones may need if disabled, it's best to learn about the options and to think about them in relation to your savings.

You can find information through AARP, the National Institute on Aging, various financial-services organizations, and others. Their websites provide tools and data that can give you ballpark estimates for different kinds of care. For example, one national survey conducted in 2016 reported that the mean annual cost of assisted living in the United States was $43,000.[5] Care for a year in a private room of a nursing home was $92,000. While such information could be useful, it's hard to compare it to the expense of staying in your own home because much of the "cost" of doing so is often borne in unpaid services provided by family and friends.

It may also be helpful to know about the government-sponsored and private agencies that help older people stay in their own homes as long as possible. Senior centers and local Area Agency on Aging offices can usually help elders to assess their needs and get assistance with in-home services such as personal care, meals, money management, home health care, transportation, and so on. Seniors pay out of pocket for some of these services, but others are free. Some are covered by Medicare or other insurance, while others are not.

One thing I've realized in observing people make these arrangements for so many years: sometimes the best solutions are the most unexpected. I have seen elderly people open their homes to relatives or roommates who provide services in exchange for rent. I have heard of groups of elderly siblings or friends who came together to share the expense of drop-in or live-in caregivers. There are people who form "pocket communities," purchasing or renting homes near each other so they can keep a watchful eye, share meals, trade chores, and so on. Of course, in designing such arrangements, we need to be vigilant and protect elderly people from those who might take advantage of their vulnerability. Still, I believe opportunities for cooperation and community building among caring, ethical people are plenty. Could it be that boomers could lead another epochal change in how we care for each other as we age? I think it could happen.

And while it makes sense to plan as best you can, it's also good to keep your mind and heart open to new situations and relationships. I'm thinking of one ACT study participant in particular. He was an elderly man of Norwegian descent who employed a Somali woman to care for him and his wife in their home during his wife's extended illness. The caregiver and the man formed a close bond and she stayed on following the wife's death. Eventually he invited the caregiver's extended family to move in as well, along with their traditional ways.

Visiting the home, I was impressed by the close, loving relationship between the couple, especially given their cultural differences. I was also nearly dumbstruck when I saw the Somali woman's cooking methods. She prepared single-pot meals in a clay vessel over an open fire in his front yard. The scene was unexpected—like something out of a *National Geographic* spread on the Horn of Africa—and certainly not a common sight in the upscale suburb of Mercer Island. I also noted how peaceful the man, the caregiver, and her family members seemed. Who could have predicted that their lives would evolve like this? I don't think anybody involved expected this outcome, but they were content and seemed very happy.

BUILDING INTENTIONAL COMMUNITIES

Among the types of places in which to grow old, one model emerges that may be particularly appealing to boomers with activist leanings. It's cohousing, a type of residential development that emphasizes social interaction while allowing residents to maintain their privacy. As one enthusiast described it, senior cohousing is "aging in community versus aging in place."

In cohousing, members actively collaborate in planning, developing, and managing a community focused on shared values and activities. The model is based on a Danish concept popularized by architects Charles Durrett and Kathryn McCamant with their 1994 book *Cohousing: A Contemporary Approach to Housing Ourselves.* The authors updated the idea for the retirement set in 2005 with *Senior Cohousing: A Community Approach to Independent Living—the Handbook.*

Typically financed like a condominium, cohousing households own their own residential units but jointly share ownership of a common house and land. The community's physical layout encourages interaction. For example, front doors and porches may face common areas; walkways lead people to naturally cross each other's paths.

While most cohousing developments are intergenerational, some have been built exclusively for people over age fifty or fifty-five. Designed with aging in mind, these communities typically have smaller units and space for live-in caregivers. Also, they explicitly define their approach to aging "in community." For example, residents may state they'll share tasks like shopping, meal preparation, and housework, but not personal care such as bathing and home health services.

But whether or not communities set age restrictions, cohousing allows older people to avoid institutional care for longer than might be possible in many conventional single-family neighborhoods, according to a policy brief from AARP.[6] Older residents benefit both from the community's social activities and from the physical security of living close to friendly neighbors.

Intergenerational cohousing communities have distinct advantages, as Sheila Hoffman, sixty-seven, and her husband, Spencer Beard, sixty-four, are finding out. The pair helped establish Capitol Hill Urban Cohousing (CHUC), a community that opened in 2016 in a densely populated Seattle neighborhood just east of downtown. Spencer and

Sheila are the only retirement-age people in the nine-family organiza-tion, and they see that as a plus.

"I did not want to be stuck in a group that's just slowing down," said Sheila, a graphic designer. Raised on the East Coast, she saw lots of her parents' generation move to traditional retirement communities in South Florida. "'God's waiting room' they call it. That's just not where Spencer and I saw ourselves headed."[7]

Instead, the couple chose an intentional community populated by people of all ages. "*Intention* is the key word," said Sheila. "Our com-munity has a shared vision and values that we developed together. Peo-ple are here because they want to be connected."

Like most cohousing communities, CHUC residents make a lot of decisions together—everything from home-financing policies to what kind of patio furniture to buy. "If you live in a retirement community with a bunch of people the same age, you're not going to have as much diversity in views," Sheila explained. But the younger people see things differently, she added. "Living here is going to challenge Spencer and me and keep our brains more engaged, I think. It's going to keep us more young and alive."

A retired elementary school physical education teacher, Spencer en-joys spending time with the children in the community. So far, two kids have learned to ride their bicycles on his watch.

He and Sheila don't have any children of their own. "But I was raised in a family with seven children, so I've got lots of kid energy," he said.[8] Last school year, the couple committed to walking one of the second-graders to her weekly after-school ballet class. And they babysit others from time to time. Such favors are sure to earn the couple "social capital" if not "surrogate grandparent" status, they believe.

"It's like extended family," Sheila said. "As Spencer and I get older and it gets more difficult for us to do things for ourselves, we hope someone will be around to say, 'Hey, can I get you anything from the store?' Or, 'Do you need a ride to the doctor next week?'"

They don't expect hands-on care from community members—that would be above and beyond. But they do plan to share their advance directives with their neighbors in case such information is needed in a medical emergency.

"There's no contract, no guarantees" that their neighbors will step up, Spencer added. But even among biological families, expectations of support sometimes go unfulfilled, they pointed out. In any community, all we can do is keep showing up with a strong intention to help and hope that others will do the same. Cohousing gives people lots of opportunities to do just that.

CONNECTING ACROSS THE GENERATIONS

As Sheila and Spencer's experience shows, reaching across generations for social reserves can be satisfying and valuable to the parties involved, as well as to the entire community. I remember back in medical school hearing renowned cultural anthropologist Margaret Mead speak about the significance of multigenerational communities. Her description of mutually beneficial relationships among children and grandparents in various cultures made a lot of sense to me. The children provide the social stimulation old folks need, while the elders give kids the stability and reliable attention they require. Meanwhile, the "sandwich generation"—those working parents who are most able to provide material support for both ends of the family—get some relief. The result is an efficient "economy."

I recently saw this dynamic during a visit to the cattle ranch that's been in my family for six generations—the place where my mother was raised. There are not a lot of high-quality childcare options out in the high country of rural Montana. So my boomer cousin Rick and his wife, Gayle, take charge of their grandchildren while Rick and Gayle's daughter and son-in-law do the work of the ranch. The little ones seem to enjoy Rick and Gayle's doting attention, and I suspect the grandparents are gaining health advantages as they meet the ever-changing challenges of caring for the ranch's next generation.

Can spending time with children help us stave off mental decline in particular? That's hard to say. But a 2016 study published in the journal of the North American Menopause Society looked into this.[9] Researchers followed 120 caregiving grandparents in Australia and found that women who babysat one day a week scored higher on cognitive tests. Grandparents may need to set their limits though; those who babysat five days a week or more had more trouble than others with cognition.

Experts in aging, education, and other human services are intrigued with the idea that strengthening intergenerational relationships can improve the lives of both elderly people and kids. In fact, many schools, churches, senior care facilities, and other institutions across the United States are experimenting with the concept.

One extraordinary example is an award-winning public charter elementary school in Cleveland, Ohio, called The Intergenerational School. It was established in 2000 by Dr. Peter J. Whitehouse and his wife, Cathy Whitehouse. Peter is my longtime friend and colleague who is a geriatric neurologist at Case Western Reserve University, and Cathy is an educator and child psychologist. The school is designed around the idea that people of all ages and abilities can productively learn together. So elders of all ages and abilities—including some with dementia—help with classroom lessons, storytelling, environmental advocacy, artwork, gardening, video games, social media, and more. This setup allows kids to get extra attention and care from the older adults—referred to as "mentors"—while the elders get the social stimulation and satisfaction of being involved in meaningful activities with kids. By 2016, the school was serving more than five hundred students—predominantly children of color who live in poverty. Hundreds of elderly mentors were involved, including many from area nursing homes. And everybody could take pride in the students' academic achievement scores; they are among the best in the nation.

The point is, every community and every family has its needs. At the same time, each person growing old can benefit by knowing their lives will continue to have meaning and purpose. One of the best ways to find happiness in old age is to contribute to the future through activities you find meaningful. Whether you're involved with kids, their parents, their schools, or any other aspect of community, helping others is a great way for you to stay resilient.

HOW LONG WILL YOU WORK?

Another important decision affecting our social well-being in aging is when to retire. It's a weighty issue that usually makes people focus carefully on finances—and for good reason. It's crucial to have enough money to live comfortably into old age.

But finances are just one part of the puzzle. We also need to think about how work affects our overall health and well-being.

For most people, employment is an important part of our identity and self-esteem. Our jobs can lend meaning, structure, and a sense of belonging to our lives. On the other hand, work can be a tremendous source of stress—especially when our jobs start to feel too physically or intellectually demanding. Dissatisfaction also comes from having too little time for pursuits that might enhance our lives as we age—things like exercise, hobbies, or spending time with loved ones. In that case, retirement can seem very appealing.

To find a balance, many boomers take a different view of work and retirement than previous generations did. Rather than seeing their mid-sixties as a hard stop to work life, they consider this time a chance to reassess their relationship to paid employment and possibly to switch gears. New approaches may range from narrowing the scope and hours of their current jobs to starting new ventures that allow for more flexibility—and hopefully more fun.

Taking a new approach makes sense when you consider the history of retirement among U.S. workers. As University of Virginia sociologist Jeff Goldsmith explains in his book *The Long Baby Boom*, the idea of retiring at age sixty-five became popular during the post–World War II manufacturing boom as unions strengthened workers' benefits and pensions. Back then, those Americans who reached age sixty-five would ultimately spend about 17 percent of their life in retirement—about 12 years. Now, that proportion is 22 percent—about 20 years—and growing. Also, about 20 percent of the workforce was engaged in physically strenuous work that could not be sustained past middle age. Today, just 8 percent of workers do hard manual labor. These days, increasingly more people are employed as knowledge workers. That is, we're laboring at computers all day—writing, designing, analyzing, programming, and so on. It's the kind of intellectually stimulating work that may actually help us sustain brain function as we age. So as long as knowledge workers can remember to get up and exercise regularly, working extra years is not likely to harm their health the way factory work may have harmed their ancestors' well-being.

Writes Dr. Goldsmith: "As knowledge work has replaced back-breaking physical labor and mind-numbing factory assembly-line work, the capacity of workers to have long careers has increased apace. Combine this with the increasing comfort workers have in mobility among firms and even among careers, and we have not only the recipe for a more flexible and adaptable labor market, but also the potential for fulfilling, serial careers."[10]

Studies indicate that most boomers are planning to work past the traditional retirement age in one way or another. A 2010 report from the Sloan Center on Aging and Work at Boston College, for example, said that 75 percent of workers aged fifty and older expected to have some kind of paid employment after retiring from their main careers.[11]

This may be a good thing given our society's need to better fund our aging population's Social Security system. Also, many boomers may need the extra earnings to fund their own needs past age sixty-five. A 2016 investment-industry research institute survey showed that just 24 percent of boomers are confident they will have enough savings for retirement. Of the 55 percent who do have retirement savings, 42 percent had less than one hundred thousand dollars, a sum that would produce less than seven thousand dollars annually in retirement income.[12]

But financial issues aside, AARP surveys show that most boomers *want* to keep working past their midsixties and would do so even if their finances did not require it.[13] The reason? They enjoy working and don't want to be bored. Perhaps many shun the idea of following in the footsteps of their parents and grandparents, who, according to Dr. Goldsmith's 2008 book, were watching forty-three hours of television a week. Indeed, over a third of those who retire in their fifties return to work within a few years, citing boredom and lack of fulfillment as a major reason, Dr. Goldsmith reported.[14]

His book provides great insight into policies that can create incentives for more flexibility toward seniors working. As of 2016, many economic, legal, and labor-related policies and practices discouraged people past age sixty-five from seeking employment options such as flex time, job sharing, phased-in retirements, consulting, sabbaticals, and so on. As Dr. Goldsmith writes, "Rather than encouraging boomers to retire, we need to revise our tax and pension policies, as well as the Social Security and Medicare programs, to encourage boomers to remain engaged, productive (and taxpaying) citizens."

HOW RETIREMENT AFFECTS HEALTH

But is employment actually better for your health than retirement? Much depends on your job conditions, of course. But for those who like their occupations, staying employed past the traditional retirement age may be beneficial, according to Drs. Milena Nikolova and Carol Graham. They are the same Brookings Institute scholars I wrote about in chapter 3—the ones who showed that people's happiness generally increases with age. In 2014, their study based on Gallup World Poll data showed that people working past retirement age were typically happier and more satisfied with their health than their retired counterparts.[15] Of course, "many of those who choose to work beyond the retirement age do so precisely because they like their work," the researchers admitted in a blog post.[16] Still, the findings provide food for thought—especially as you consider what you might want to pursue as an "encore career."

Be aware that some research points to health hazards immediately following retirement, and not just because of retirees' existing medical conditions. Rather, people often struggle with issues such as depression, weight gain, marital problems, too much alcohol, and other causes of stress after they leave work. In fact, overall death rates rise dramatically in the years immediately following retirement.[17]

Also, health risks seem to be greater for people who retire earlier than their peers. Esteban Calvo, a sociologist at Diego Portales University in Chile, is leading a longitudinal study of more than one hundred thousand people in twenty-one countries to examine the health effects of retirement. His team is looking at overall health, chronic diseases, the ability to perform daily activities, and happiness levels. Based on preliminary results, he told the *Washington Post* in 2015 that retirement has negative health effects on people who retire earlier than the mean age, and the outcomes are worse the earlier you stop working. "It's not that you have to work forever," he said. "But those who retire too early feel more sad and lonely and disconnected."[18]

Several studies comparing people across industrialized nations have also shown a strong relationship between early retirement age and diminished cognitive function.[19] For example, one large study conducted by researchers from RAND and the University of Michigan compared men in France and Austria—where fewer men in their early sixties are employed—to men in places like the United States and Denmark—where more men work past the middle sixties. The authors concluded that later employment could be the cause for better cognitive performance among the American and Danish men.[20] Another study, published in 2013 by Italian researchers from the University of Padua, found "a strong positive association between cognitive decline and years in retirement after controlling for age, physical health, income, education, and early-life conditions."[21]

HOLDING ON TO INTELLECT, MEANING, AND PURPOSE

While these studies about mental decline in retirement can be scary, please don't despair. I draw two important lessons from such research for those who want to stay mentally fit as they approach retirement age:

1. If you can keep working—and especially if you have an occupation that you find enjoyable and stimulating—go ahead and stay employed. You will probably benefit mentally and physically by keeping yourself actively engaged in your work life. This is true whether you're working for pay or as a volunteer.

2. If you'd rather retire or cut back on working, that's great too. But whatever path you take, *don't go into mental retirement.* There's great truth in the phrase "use it or lose it." You've got to continue to keep your mind actively engaged if you want to maintain your thinking skills. So as you leave your job, be sure to find meaningful new ways to keep your brain working. This requires far more than doing crossword puzzles! It means having activities that give your life structure, that challenge your mind, and that keep you socially and physically active. Such activities might include volunteer work, hobbies, sports, religious activities, or whatever. Just make it rich, and make it count.

If you decide to keep working, but want to switch gears as you approach retirement age, there are many alternatives to consider. One is to gradually narrow the scope of your job or the number of hours you're working. Perhaps you can stay in the same field but focus on the part of your work you like the best. I have known many researchers and teachers who zero in on just one subject—a move that allows them to bring new passion to their work as they age. It's a way to capitalize on their mastery at the same time they dial back the energy required.

Another approach is to switch your role from being the hands-on problem solver to being a mentor or consultant to others. This switch recognizes that we generally develop two types of intelligence in our lives. One is "fluid intelligence," which involves our current ability to deal with complex problems using abstract thinking. Although highly variable among individuals, fluid intelligence typically peaks in adolescence and may start to progressively decline in our thirties or forties. Examples might be learning cutting-edge technologies or new programming skills. The other is "crystallized intelligence," which involves knowledge that comes from prior learning and past experiences. This type of intelligence typically peaks at around age sixty to seventy. (Again, these are just averages; there's lots of variation among people.) When we take on the role of teacher or consultant to others later in our careers, we can leverage our crystallized intelligence. This can be particularly valuable in volunteer work. Many retired professionals provide tremendous service in this capacity, especially by serving on the boards of nonprofit organizations, for example.

Of course, you can also go in a completely new direction, leaving your main occupation and trying a new role, starting a new business, or pursuing some unexplored aspect of yourself. Your new pursuit can lend a whole new meaning to the idea of "bucket list." That is, instead of cataloging all the places you want to visit before you die, think of all the facets of yourself you'd like to develop. Artist? Teacher? Musician? Swimmer? Caregiver? Inventor? Environmentalist? Spiritual seeker? True friend? How about the World's Best Grandparent? The possibilities are endless.

MAKE IT MEAN SOMETHING

Whatever choices you make regarding work, volunteer service, or leisure-time activities as you grow older, here are a few basic—but very important—questions to ask:

- What activities do you find most meaningful in your life?

- What kind of work—whether paid or not paid—gives you the sense that you're contributing something important to the world?
- How will you continue to pursue meaningful activities as you grow older?

As surveys have shown, seniors feel that having a sense of purpose is important to successful aging. Knowing your purpose gets you going in the morning and keeps you engaged in the world mentally, physically, and socially. It can feed that sense of "generativity" that we explored in chapter 3—the idea that you're contributing something valuable to future generations. That could be your own family members, your neighbors, your community, or the world at large. Having a sense of purpose also helps you avoid the loneliness and listlessness that can set in if you don't have enough social interaction or structure in your days.

I know many people who made important purpose-driven shifts in their lives at age sixty-five or so. One example is Dr. Bob Zufall, whom I introduced in chapter 3. He found tremendous fulfillment in his sixties and beyond by continuing to practice medicine but shifting his focus from serving private-practice urology patients to opening a free primary care clinic for disadvantaged people in his community. Remember he found his path by asking, "What needs to be done that I *can* do and that I *enjoy* doing?"

Another example is Wendy Townsend, who was a fifty-seven-year-old marketing executive in 1999 when she found her niche in our area's senior services community. She saw that many younger people were benefiting from yoga practice, but nobody was offering "gentle yoga" classes designed for older bodies.

Wendy wasn't yet ready to leave her job as vice president of a Seattle-area credit union, so she hatched her plan in phases, as many soon-to-be retirees do. Step one was to take a year's leave of absence to get the requisite training, a move she combined with caring for her newborn grandson. She then returned to the credit union for another four years, negotiating with her employer for permission to teach a few classes during the week at area retirement communities, senior centers, and churches. So by the time Wendy was ready to fully retire from her forty-year career in marketing and public relations, she had her second career fully launched.

Now seventy-three, Wendy continues to teach six to seven yoga classes a week, including one all-ages class held Sunday evenings on the altar platform at the city's landmark Episcopal cathedral.

Over the years, she has combined her teaching with chauffeur duties for her two grandsons. Committing to pick them up after school has given her and her husband a fail-safe way to stay connected to them—something many grandparents long for but fail to achieve. Even after the boys were old enough to ride a bike or take a bus, she kept it up. "Why wouldn't you want to see your grandkids each day?" she asked. "It's such a boost!"[22]

When Wendy first started her yoga training in 1999, she was focused on teaching seniors in her mother's generation. Now she has aged into that population herself, and she's experiencing the benefits of frequent practice. She has no health problems other than some arthritis in her hips. It's likely that the muscle strength she built through yoga helped her recover quickly from her first hip replacement surgery several years ago. And she's counting on it doing the same when she gets the other hip joint replaced soon.

Wendy also benefits from knowing that people expect her to show up every day. She is a lot like the seniors in Evangeline Shuler's retirement community who met for coffee every single morning, rain or shine. They did it for themselves, and they did it for each other.

"The motivation to be with others is what gets me out of bed," said Wendy. "I know I have to go meet this person, or teach that class, or pick up my grandson. It just feels good to know that people are counting on me."

It's an attitude that comes from her proactive approach, her acceptance of the aging process, and her work to build reserves—mentally, physically, and socially.

8

CHOOSE YOUR OWN ENDING

Your Reward for a Life Well Lived

In previous chapters you met great role models for resilience in old age. You've seen how people get activated to take good care of their health. You've learned how they accept the inevitable changes that come with age, and how they build the mental, physical, and social reserves to cultivate well-being.

To what end? Ideally, you come to a place where you can relax and grow very old, knowing you're safe, comfortable, and well cared for.

My patient Rolando Perez, introduced in chapter 7, had come to that place at age ninety-nine. His hearing, vision, and short-term memory were failing, but otherwise he was in pretty good shape. He still lived contentedly in his own home—thanks in large part to the caring relationships and mutual devotion within his large family. And by all accounts, he still enjoyed his life.

Although I was Rolando's primary care doctor in his later years, I didn't see him as often as you might think. He had reached the stage where he needed what I call "late-in-life" care. This is not to be confused with "end-of-life" care, which nowadays is often delivered by a hospice team following a terminal diagnosis.

In contrast, late-in-life care is for elderly people who are essentially well but getting on in years—say, age eighty-five and up. Because of their advanced age, they may need extra attention from family, friends, and care providers. For example, an annual flu shot is warranted, along with treatments to relieve annoying or troublesome symptoms of chronic conditions such as arthritis, anemia, or skin problems. Antibiotics for acute trouble such as a urinary tract infection make sense.

But there are many kinds of care that very elderly people absolutely don't need—and that might actually be harmful to them. That's because too much health care can upset homeostasis—that delicate sense of internal stability I described in chapter 3 that often keeps very old people active in those last precious years. Most frail elderly people don't need the stress of colonoscopies, mammograms, Pap smears, PSA blood tests, and other diagnostic procedures aimed at finding cancers, the treatment of which few would survive.

Nor would I necessarily recommend surgery for nonmelanoma skin cancer, which predominantly affects older people. Having surgery to remove such lesions can result in complications related to wound healing, numbness, and pain. Since such lesions don't typically affect survival or long-term quality of life for the elderly, it makes more sense to leave most of these lesions alone.

Also, frail people don't need drugs that put them at risk for falls and foggy thinking. This includes many medications for high blood pressure, anxiety, trouble sleeping, or incontinence. And the last thing they need is an unnecessary trip to urgent care or the hospital emergency department, where they might be subjected to a battery of high-tech medical tests and interventions, causing them stress and confusion from which they might never recover.

So unlike many elderly people whose lives seem to revolve around medical appointments and hospital stays, Rolando came to see me at the clinic every one to two years. In between visits, his daughter and I discussed his care via phone calls and email, adjusting his medications as needed to treat his diabetes and other chronic conditions. This allowed him to spend his time the way he preferred, watching his favorite TV game shows and taking slow walks to the grocery store for lottery tickets. Why visit the doctor's office when you can get your grandson to take you to a casino?

Eventually, though, Rolando's immune system and everyday defense mechanisms grew more diminished. In July 2012, he caught a cold but was no longer able to produce a strong cough. This led to pneumonia. Antibiotics cleared this lung infection, but afterward his daughters sensed his end was near. His energy was waning, and he stopped coming downstairs for breakfast.

By September "he would not eat anything," Rebecca Perez remembers.[1] His daughters tried feeding him, "but he would just spit it out." Rebecca and Barbara began taking turns staying in his room at night. "We wanted to be sure that if he had to get up, he didn't fall," explained Barbara.[2] "We would be there to watch."

"One night he woke up and said, 'Mama . . . Mama . . .' like a premonition—like he thought somebody was coming to pick him up," Rebecca recalled.

And on the morning of Monday, October 8, that ride arrived. He had been particularly restless from midnight on. Around dawn, Rolando told Rebecca, "We have to go," and he struggled to get up. Rebecca helped him into the chair next to his bed.

"He asked for the old woolen cap he liked to wear when he was cold," Rebecca said. "So I put it on him." Then, about 7 a.m., this very old and very well-loved man stopped breathing and died.

His daughters called the priest from St. Benedict's, who came to offer a blessing over Rolando's remains. Finding him sitting up with his ski cap in place, the priest commented, "He certainly looks like he was ready for the trip."

WHAT IS A "GOOD DEATH"?

It may seem strange, or even insensitive, to suggest that Rolando's death was "ideal." His family grieved his passing and the emptiness it left in their hearts and their community. Still, his daughters knew he had lived a good, long life, and they were glad to be with him when he died peacefully in his own home. After so many years of helping others, it seemed fitting that he would experience his last days like this—as though a good death truly was his reward for a life well lived.

From my conversations with patients about end-of-life wishes, I know Rolando's passing was the kind many people wish for. He was not in pain. He was not alone. He was not angry or confused. He was not in the hospital connected to tubes and wires. And he did not linger.

According to public surveys and research studies, this is the way 80 percent of Americans would like to go; they want to be at home and avoid high-intensity care and hospitalization.[3] Unfortunately, in today's world of high-tech, life-extending medicine and far-flung family relationships, death too rarely comes in the quiet, humane way that it arrived for Rolando Perez. A study of more than 840,000 who died while covered by fee-for-service Medicare showed that use of intensive care in the last month of life increased from 24.3 percent in 2000 to 29.2 percent in 2005 and 2009.[4]

What can be done to make a so-called good death experience more common? That's a question doctors, clergy, researchers, policy makers, and patients are asking with more frequency—especially as aging boomers experience their parents' deaths and anticipate their own. And just as boomers did with hot-button issues in our youth (think the Vietnam War, the women's movement), our generation now brings an activated sensibility to this last stage of life. We are, after all, the cohort that pressed Western society on reproductive freedom, home-style and alternative birthing practices, shared decision making in medicine, and countless other forms of patient-centered health care. Now, as boomers anticipate making similar demands in care for the dying, more care providers, patients, and their families are engaging in conversations about patients' individual preferences and values regarding care at the end of life.

Still, these conversations are not easy, especially when there may be as many variations on "a good death" as there are people dying. One group exploring these issues—especially from the patient's perspective—is led by Dilip Jeste, director of the Sam and Rose Stein Institute for Research on Aging at the University of California, San Diego School of Medicine. His team published a paper in the *American Journal of Geriatric Psychiatry* in 2016 that reviewed academic articles on what constitutes a good death—according to people who are dying, their relatives, and health care providers.[5] Dr. Jeste's team is collecting this information to help identify the unmet needs of dying people and to find ways to make their care more individualized. This work acknowledges that society can't promise people a "good death" unless we can find better ways to talk about it.

You'd think there would be plenty of literature at hand. But in fact the team looked in the massive PubMed and PsychINFO databases and found only thirty-six articles published between 1996 and 2015 that met their inclusion and quality criteria. They used these to surface definitions of "successful dying" and then categorized them into the following themes, each with "subthemes" listed in parentheses:

- Preferences for the dying process (determining how death will occur, who will be there, where, and when; dying in sleep; and making preparations such as advance directives and funeral arrangements)
- Pain-free status (not suffering; having pain and symptom management)
- Emotional well-being (getting emotional support; psychological comfort; having a chance to discuss the meaning of death)
- Family (having family support, family accepting of death, family prepared for death, not being a burden to the family)
- Dignity (being respected as an individual and maintaining independence)
- Life completion (saying good-bye, feeling that life was well lived, and accepting impending death)
- Religiosity/spirituality (religious or spiritual comfort; faith; meeting with clergy)
- Treatment preferences (not prolonging life, a belief that all available treatments were used; control of treatment; accessing euthanasia/physician-assisted death)
- Quality of life (living life as usual; maintaining hope, pleasure, gratitude; feeling life is worth living)
- Relationship with health care provider (having trust in and gaining support and comfort from physicians and nurses; having a physician who is comfortable with death and dying; being able to discuss spiritual beliefs or fears with a physician)
- Other (recognition of culture; experiencing physical touch; being with pets; considering health care costs)

Dr. Jeste's team then determined the frequency with which each group (patients, family members, and care providers) mentioned these themes. It's interesting to consider the similarities and differences among the groups regarding what each felt was important. For example, honoring patients' preferences, staying pain free, and having emotional well-being were highly regarded across all groups. Groups differed, however, regarding quality of life, which was mentioned as important by 70 percent of the family member reports but just 35 percent of the patient reports and 22 percent of the health care worker reports. Life completion, dignity, and presence of the family were noted more frequently in family member perspectives than in patient perspectives. And the patients' reports referred to religiosity/spirituality more often than family member reports did.

"For a dying person, the concerns seem to be more existential and psychological and less physical," Dr. Jeste told reporters after his review was published.[6] His team acknowledged that health care systems need to attend to the dying patient's physical needs—such as pain control—but providers also need to "address the psychological, social, and religiosity/spirituality themes in end-of-life care for both patients and families."

This advice makes sense—especially as our society begins caring for a burgeoning population of elderly people who have a rich history of upsetting social norms. Who can predict how far boomers—with their high interest in autonomy and freedom of choice—might challenge what's considered acceptable in care for the dying? One obvious example is the rapidly evolving legal framework addressing physician-assisted death. By 2016, physician-assisted death under certain circumstances was legal in Oregon, Washington, Montana, and California—covering about 16 percent of the U.S. population. Change toward allowing gravely ill patients more aid in dying was underway in other states too—as well as in Canada and other countries around the world.

What does such a sea change mean for our society as aging boomers grow old and die over the next few decades? One thing is likely: you will be asked with increasing frequency to speak up about the kinds of care you want—and don't want—in the run-up to your inevitable passing. I hope you'll have had a chance to reflect on your expectations, your fears, your wishes, and your values. And I hope you'll have a good death, however you define it.

But ultimately, the only person who can help you decide how you want to live your last days and finally to die is you. And—as many well know—our thoughts and feelings about dying are greatly influenced by having cared for our own relatives and dear friends at the times of their deaths.

OUR PARENTS, OURSELVES

Architect Paul Leland, age fifty-six, told me how the death of his elderly parents influenced his own ideas about choices he hopes to make at the end of his life. He was struck by the stark difference in his father's and mother's experiences. His father died in an Omaha hospital intensive care unit after days of unsuccessful intervention; his mom died peacefully in her sleep at his sister's home.

"I saw how you just can't predict how circumstances might play out for you," Paul said.[7] "And I learned that there comes a point when—no matter how strong your medical team and your will to live—modern medicine gives way to old age and frailty."

That's how it was for Paul's father, Tom Leland, the tough-minded eighty-nine-year-old ex-cop I wrote about in chapter 4 who had battled heart disease and diabetes for nearly four decades. Although he still had his sense of humor and enjoyed being with his wife and family, his life had been limited for many years by chronic illness, joint pain, and depression. He also suffered from mild dementia, likely caused by small strokes.

So when his dad landed in the hospital with a bowel obstruction, Paul was worried but not surprised. This had happened repeatedly due to scar tissue in his intestines from a previous surgery. Usually it resolved with time and minimal treatment. Only this time, the blockage was not resolving and the family faced a tough decision. Tom could have surgery to clear the obstruction, but keeping his lungs clear during the procedure would be difficult. If they failed to do so, there was a high risk of life-threatening pneumonia. And what if their dad didn't have the surgery? He would surely die.

Because of Tom's dementia, the surgeon turned to Paul for a decision. As his dad's proxy for health care, Paul knew that Tom had created an "advance directive"—the legal form that patients complete to describe their wishes for care. Tom's directive stated that he did not want to be kept alive by artificial means if there was no hope for survival. But how was the family to interpret that direction in this situation? What were the chances Tom could beat the odds? What if the surgery was successful and he didn't develop pneumonia? Paul knew his dad was a fighter who had tremendous confidence in his doctors. That had worked for him in the past under circumstances that seemed more dire than this. He also knew his dad had a strong religious faith; Tom was not one to give up on hope for staying alive. This made Paul think his father would want to go for it. So he went to his dad's bedside and asked him if he wanted to have the operation, even with its risks. Though somewhat bewildered, the old man said yes.

Tom survived the surgery, but in the days that followed, his condition deteriorated just as the surgeon warned it might. Contents of his stomach had gotten into his lungs when Tom was under anesthesia, introducing bacteria that developed into pneumonia. To breathe, he was placed on a mechanical ventilator with a tube in his mouth pumping oxygen into his windpipe. Unable to move or communicate, he became increasingly confused and agitated. He tried to pull out the breathing tube, the heart monitors, the urinary catheter, and the IV. Tom's children took turns at his bedside in the intensive care unit. They passed hours holding down his arms, futilely trying to keep him from tugging on the equipment. And when they could no longer stop him, the staff tied their father's arms to his bed.

"It was heartbreaking to see our dad struggle like that," says Paul. He and his siblings remember their dad as the strong, vibrant character he was before he got sick. As a younger man, he had served in the navy and coached Little League baseball. He loved to fix old cars, sing like Hank Williams, and take his four kids fishing and camping. These memories of him could not be diminished by his illnesses and this awful struggle in his final hours—and yet that image stays with them.

Within two days, it became clear that Tom's lungs were not going to recover. The family agreed it was time to take him off the ventilator. For comfort, the nurses replaced it with an external oxygen pump that forced air into his nose. Over the next twenty-four hours, Tom lost consciousness and his lungs slowly stopped working.

"Thinking back, I see that my father died in a way that was consistent with his values," Paul said. "He was a fighter and a believer, and he lived that way to the end." But Paul also acknowledged that if the family had truly understood the risks of the surgery and could have predicted the suffering that would occur in its aftermath, they might have made a different choice. It's in instances like these that accepting the limitations of modern medicine and the reality of death can be a blessing.

As a physician, I know how hard it is to communicate these realities to patients and their families when lives are on the line. But once you've watched your parent die a difficult death in an ICU—or even worse, linger on a ventilator while family members vacillate over what to do— you have a much deeper understanding of the trade-offs. Unfortunately, Tom's experience is not uncommon. And that's why I believe his children's generation, now in their fifties and sixties, may approach their own deaths better equipped with a more complete understanding for making choices about their own end-of-life care.

Paul's memory of his father's arduous passing is tempered by knowledge of how his mother died just three years later. Dorothy also suffered from dementia, although the cause was unknown. A CT scan taken after a fall when she was eighty-five years old showed lesions on her brain suspected to be cancer. But Dorothy was already frail, so Paul's family agreed with her doctor that there was no point in doing further diagnostic work. For one, a definitive imaging test would require Dorothy to ingest a liquid that might damage her aging kidneys. And even if brain cancer was confirmed, she was too frail to survive treatment. So she lived another five years, becoming increasingly weak and demented. Taking care of her was not easy. By the end, she could no longer walk and needed help twenty-four hours a day. But she did not suffer unnecessary surgeries and medical treatment. And her final days were peaceful ones, spent at home with family and caregivers, who had the support of a hospice care team.

THE LIMITS OF ADVANCE DIRECTIVES

Most people believe that creating a legal document called an "advance directive" will make care decisions easier at the end of life. Even before Congress passed the Patient Self-Determination Act in 1990, which made the practice standard, I urged my patients to complete such documents and share them with their relatives and health care teams. I had witnessed too many situations where patients suffered a "bad death" because doctors, nurses, and family members simply did not know what a gravely ill person wanted. And uncertainty almost always leads to prolonged and often agonizing care of no value.

Advance directives, which include "living wills" and durable powers of attorney for health care, allow people to accept or reject care and to appoint others to make care decisions for them if they are no longer able. According to the national Health and Retirement Study, by 2010, 72 percent of Americans over age sixty had created advance directives, up from 47 percent in 2000.[8]

But, as many families have discovered, simply creating an advance directive does not help in all decision-making situations concerning late-life or end-of-life care. Related problems are varied and plenty. For many, the language used is both too vague and outmoded to be practical. (At what point does a condition become "terminal"? How long is "a persistent vegetative state"?)

Sometimes people complete an advance directive and then stash it in a file without telling their relatives or health care teams. Or they give it to their doctor and then it gets lost in the massive medical records patients can accumulate. Some health systems include advance directives in electronic health records, but others do not. And some electronic health record systems alert doctors that an advance directive is on file but the doctor can't get to the contents of the document when needed.

In a typical scenario, the patient turns up in the emergency room to be cared for by doctors who don't know the advance directive exists. With the patient incapacitated, the provider turns to next of kin for direction, but relatives can only guess what Mom or Dad would want. It's surprising how often families are caught off guard by the final crisis of their loved one's long life. And sometimes, in the heat of such a crisis, the patient's instructions simply get overridden. The traumatized spouse or adult child of the patient has just one focused request: keep my loved one alive.

That's how it was for Nance Reichmann in 2015 when she called an ambulance for her husband Carl. At ninety-one, the retired California building contractor had been in good health. He was an avid fisherman and world traveler with no serious medical problems. In fact, he and Nance were making plans to take a cruise in the next few months. But one night in late December—when most of their family was away in Florida—Carl simply fell ill.

It started with pain in his legs. By the next morning, he was too weak to get out of bed. Panicked, Nance called 911. Once at the hospital, Carl went immediately to the ICU, where the doctor said he was gravely ill with pneumonia and the infection was causing his vital organs to shut down. Treatment would require strong IV antibiotics. He would also need a ventilator to breathe.

Did Nance think about Carl's advance directive at that moment? "Probably not," said Dana Meyers, their granddaughter who relayed the story to me.[9] Nance's husband of sixty-nine years was suddenly and inexplicably dying. She wanted the doctor to do everything possible to save his life.

"Miraculously, the antibiotics worked and he came back from the pneumonia," Dana recalled. But by the time Carl was out of the woods he had been on the ventilator for about three weeks and could no longer breathe without it. In the meantime, Carl could not eat or drink. He was getting all his nutrition through a tube in his stomach. For comfort, the doctors performed a tracheotomy, an incision in his neck that allowed the breathing tube to be placed directly into Carl's windpipe. Then Carl was moved to a rehab facility to begin "weaning" him off the ventilator. Carl's therapy continued for two months, a process Dana describes as "one step forward, two steps back."

"His mind was still fully there, but because of the tracheotomy, he could not talk," she said. "So he would write on a piece of paper or we would try to read his lips. . . . Still, he was completely with it. He was a giant presence in the room, and he wanted to take care of everybody else."

By mid-March, however, Carl was still not breathing on his own and his doctors regretfully told his family that they did not believe he ever would. In the meantime, complications with the feeding tube had made it difficult for him to get nutrition for several days. As Carl grew weaker and less alert, his family came to understand the implications: this was exactly what Carl, in his advance directive, said he did not want—to be kept alive by artificial means. And because he could no longer communicate his own wishes, Nance and her children had to make the decision for him. It was excruciating, but eventually they knew that it was time for the doctor to order "terminal care." On March 25, the nurse administered a large dose of IV morphine, enough to cause Carl to lose consciousness, so that he would not suffer when the breathing machine was removed. Within a few hours, Carl was gone.

Dana says her grandmother endured many difficult moments throughout Carl's ordeal, from first learning his condition was grave, to his grueling rehab therapy, to saying good-bye before the nurse removed the ventilator. "But she said the hardest part was making these choices. She said if he had just died of a heart attack, that would have been so painful, but she would not have had to make all of these diffi-cult decisions."

Carl's story reminds me of an adage, "Pneumonia is a friend of the elderly." This was true years ago, before drugs and technology could keep elderly people with weak defense mechanisms alive longer than nature would otherwise allow. Back then, as now, pneumonia was con-sidered a relatively humane way for old people to die. Today, when we prolong life by artificial means, we must ask, how much time and what quality of life are patients gaining? We may expect to address the issue by creating advance directives. But this process is often undone in real-world circumstances such as Carl's, where an acute illness happens suddenly and mysteriously, complicating decision making; family mem-bers may cling to hope rather than follow a document based on ima-gined circumstances that don't resemble the crisis before them.

Even with the limitations of advance directives, my advice to every-one is this: do complete such documentation spelling out your wishes, and name someone—a close friend or family member—to make deci-sions for you if you become incapacitated. It's an important step for all adults to take, no matter what your age or physical condition. (As Carl's family discovered, illness or injury can strike at any time, so it's best to be prepared.)

Having an up-to-date advance care plan is especially important when you have a life-limiting illness that could affect your ability to make decisions on your own behalf in the near future. Examples include advanced cancer, heart failure, end-stage COPD, stroke, and Alzhei-mer's disease. Or when many functions start to fail, even without a specific illness or injury.

And remember, an advance care plan is only that—a plan. In addi-tion to documentation, we need real conversations with our physicians, other caregivers, relatives, and friends to inform our decisions.

Help to frame such conversations is available from organizations such as Compassion & Choices (www.compassionandchoices.org) and Aging with Dignity (www.agingwithdignity.org). Both provide compre-hensive guides to help people explore their values and develop the right legal documents to describe their wishes. They also provide tools for talking about end-of-life care with your family, friends, and health care providers.

Once you fill out the forms and work with the tools, tell others about the choices you've made. That's really the best way to make it likely that they'll follow your wishes.

PHYSICIANS WANT TO HELP

Although much can be done to make advance care planning better, we have come a long way. I remember how doctors and patients talked about death when I was a resident in internal medicine in the early seventies. Although my colleagues and I may have had private conversations with families about "helping someone to die" by providing large doses of narcotics, there were no formal protocols like we have today for patients with terminal illness. Modern hospice programs, designed explicitly to provide good quality of care and comfort to the dying, were nonexistent in the United States back then. In fact, before the hospice movement of the 1970s, it was common and acceptable for doctors to conceal from dying patients their terminal status. In many cases, doctors didn't even reveal to a terminal patient's family that their loved one was likely to die soon. I think most would agree that reversing medicine's paternalistic attitudes toward death has made today's end-of-life care more humane. But for many doctors and patients, talking openly about dying and making decisions for end-of-life care is still a challenge.

Efforts to improve this are under way. Congress passed legislation in 2016 allowing Medicare to reimburse doctors for time spent discussing advance care planning with patients in outpatient settings. While that's a major step in the right direction, additional solutions are needed. In 2015, a committee from the Institute of Medicine released a report called *Dying in America: Improving Quality and Honoring Individual Preferences near the End of Life*.[10] It concluded that the U.S. health care system is poorly designed to meet the needs of patients and their families. The committee called for "standards for clinician-patient communication and advance care planning that are measurable, actionable, and evidence-based." It recommended major changes to the way we educate and train doctors, as well as changes in practice, policy, and payment systems. Writing in the *New England Journal of Medicine*, committee cochairs Philip A. Pizzo and David M. Walker also called for radical reforms in individual and public education to promote more meaningful discussions between patients and clinicians about end-of-life planning.[11]

To address the obstacles physicians face, the Hartford Foundation and others conducted a nationwide survey in 2016 of 736 primary care doctors and specialists—all of whom see patients aged sixty-five and over.[12] The survey showed that virtually all the doctors said they consider end-of-life and advance care planning conversations important. And most said they believe they—not the patient or another health care professional—are responsible for starting these dialogues. But nearly half reported that they frequently feel unsure about what to say.

What gets in the way? The doctors in the survey pointed to health system barriers, such as having no formal way to assess patients' wishes and goals. They also cited problems getting access to patients' advance care plans via electronic health records. And most felt that doctors need better training in how to lead discussions with their patients. Those surveyed who had received explicit coaching expressed more confidence about having such conversations and were more likely to find these talks "rewarding."

Importantly, a vast majority of the doctors surveyed see advance care planning as a way to honor the patient's values and wishes, reduce unwanted hospitalizations at the end of life, and have patients and families feel more satisfied with their care. Still, such conversations are not easy. About half the doctors said they were concerned that their patient might feel they were "giving up" on them or that the conversation could cause the patients themselves "to give up hope."

ARE WE REALLY "AT WAR" WITH DEATH?

Do patients see advance care planning as a sign of surrender? If the Hartford Foundation survey is correct, that seems to be what doctors fear. One problem may be our society's tendency to frame medicine as a battleground. If we're engaged in a "war against cancer" or a "fight against heart disease," perhaps we can think of death only in terms of defeat. Thus modern medicine avoids "failure" by promoting an illusion that patients can successfully pursue every high-tech intervention and magic-bullet treatment at all costs. This bias toward high-tech intervention, unchecked, harms many patients and families near the end of life, robbing them of quality time and peace of mind. It causes patients to cling to expectations that their doctors will act with urgency to "do something" in every instance—whether or not that "something" can help. I see this often in the care of patients with Alzheimer's disease, a condition that tragically lacks few, if any, effective treatments that modify the course of the illness. Despite this, families don't want to foreclose on hope, so they press for any treatment at all—even knowing there's little chance of improvement. They just want to be assured they've done all they can for their loved one.

It's as though we believe humanity can conquer aging in the same way we learned to beat back infectious disease or heal the traumatic injuries of war. But the chronic conditions of late life are different from polio, gunshot wounds, or broken bones. Aging is not "cured" with antibiotics, great surgical technique, or even gene therapy. Given that there's no way to win the "battle" against aging, perhaps we need a new metaphor for health care near the end of life—one that buries the hatchet and puts doctors, patients, and the true nature of life and death all on the same side.

Any progress in this direction will surely be rooted in the wisdom of Elisabeth Kubler-Ross, the Swiss-born psychiatrist who published *On Death and Dying* in 1969.[13] Noting that medical school curricula weren't teaching doctors about such topics, Dr. Kubler-Ross interviewed dying patients at the University of Chicago medical school as the basis of her studies. As a young medical student, I vividly remember how her book and seminars affected me—especially her widely acclaimed theory on the "stages of grief" that people experience as they face their impending deaths. Her work opened a door to better understanding dying people's needs and offered insights that allow us to help patients find meaning and acceptance in their experience. Dr. Kubler-Ross also legitimized end-of-life care as an important area for research. However, it was not until the hospice movement of the 1970s that our society truly seemed to begin accepting the limitations of treatment for some conditions, especially advanced cancers, and helping people to prepare for death.

With the help of hospice providers who excel at palliative care (also known as "comfort care"), most patients with such terminal illnesses and their families can get the support needed to avoid unnecessary treatment, and they're having better outcomes as a result. A 2010 study of patients with lung cancer showed that early palliative care led to significant improvements in both quality of life and mood.[14] When researchers compared these patients to a similar group receiving standard care, they found that, despite receiving less aggressive care at the end of life, those with palliative care actually had longer survival.

But palliative care and hospice programs are not enough. A similar approach is needed for older people before they develop serious illnesses and terminal conditions so they too can sidestep overdiagnosis and overtreatment. Our society needs a more standard approach to such "late-in-life" care because treatment of many common conditions becomes riskier and more complicated as we grow older. Also, late-in-life patients almost always experience less benefit from treatment than younger patients do. Cancer therapies, for example, are more challenging in elderly patients because they have fewer reserves to withstand the assaults of radiation, chemotherapy, and surgery. Also, the older person's weakened immunity makes them more vulnerable to infections.

Elderly people undergoing major surgery face increased risks that can shorten their lives or adversely affect the quality of their lives going forward. Anesthesia and operations in general, for example, can put older minds at risk for short-term delirium and long-term dementia. I remember one of my patients in his early eighties who had a sharp mind but needed coronary bypass surgery. Other than his age, he seemed strong and well suited for the operation. Afterward, however, he suffered from delirium and never fully recovered his brain function. Cases like these, both in my practice and documented in scientific literature, have convinced me that if you want to live long with high quality of life, when it comes to health care, less is often more.

WHICH WAY TO THE EXIT?

And what happens when illness or frailty so diminish the quality of your life that you're ready to die? Most people would agree this would be a good time for death to take us. If we're lucky, we may be like Rolando Perez. We'll live happily to age ninety-nine, have a premonition that death is coming, put on a traveling hat, and wait just a few minutes for the ride to arrive.

Maybe that's what Evangeline Shuler had in mind when, at age 107, she engaged her physician grandson in a frank request about her desired exit. Having fallen and broken her pelvis eight months earlier, she could no longer stand or walk, much less dance her beloved tango.

"We got her out of bed three times a day to come to the table and eat with us," recalled Van's daughter Lynn, with whom she lived in Florida.[15] "She seemed to enjoy that." But eventually Van chose to spend most of her days in bed.

Lynn remembered Van's exchange with her grandson. "She asked him, 'Without bothering you, without hurting you legally, do you have anything to give me to help me to die?' But he told her, 'No, Grandma, doctors are trained not to do that. We have an oath to keep people alive.' So that was that."

Weeks passed as Evangeline waited patiently, unable to see, unable to feed herself, and barely able to move on her own. Eventually, in 2014 at the age of 108, she passed away.

Physicians who work with terminally ill patients and the very old would not be surprised to hear of Evangeline's request to her grandson. They know that people reach a point where they no longer resist death but see it as an inevitable next step on their journey. They've also encountered patients of all ages who wish to take control of their destiny, and so they ask their doctors for help in dying.

My own ideas about helping patients to die have evolved over time. When I was a young physician, I thought I knew better than my patients did what they needed. And still today, if I think somebody is making a choice about dying based on inadequate knowledge of what the future could hold for them, I will let them know. They may not understand, for example, that their condition or their state of mind could improve, and if they wait, they might make a different choice. But if I know that a patient has a solid grasp of their situation and feels that their illness or disability is making a meaningful life impossible, my guiding principle is to respect that person's autonomy in choosing whether to live or die.

It's my sense that a growing number of people want such autonomy—especially as more and more boomers face life-threatening illnesses and disability. (Would we expect anything less from the generation that exercised such a rebellious streak at every other major life transition?) An increasing number of health care providers can now accommodate patient's requests for help in dying, as more states and countries pass laws allowing physician-assisted death. In Washington State, where I practice, patients have had legal access to physician-assisted death since 2008.

Opponents of such laws worry that families or institutions might pressure patients to end their lives because of the burden or cost of caring for them. But the state laws have strong safeguards in place that, thus far, seem to be preventing any such exploitation. These include requiring a waiting period between the times a patient requests and receives the lethal dose of barbiturate medication to hasten death. Patients must also show proof that they are mentally competent, not suffering from a mental illness, and have a life expectancy of no more than six months. In Washington and Oregon, physicians who provide the drug are required to report every case to the state or the law won't protect them.

Although some see these provisions as burdensome, I believe they're important because they address a fundamental truth about the human condition: death is a one-way passage. Once an individual accepts society's aid for their journey, there is no turning back. Therefore, we must do our absolute best to ensure that each person choosing physician-aided death does so with a sound mind, clear resolve, and without pressure from others. We don't want to risk that people make the irreversible decision for aid in dying when treatment or even watchful waiting might be a better alternative.

To date, relatively few people have chosen to use the assisted-death provision. For example, Oregon, which implemented its law in 1997, saw an increase in reports of physician-assisted death from 0.5 in 1,000 deaths in 1998 to 3.86 in 1,000 deaths in 2015. More people request the medication than actually take it. Among the 218 patients for whom lethal prescriptions were written in Oregon in 2015, just 125 (57.3 percent) took the medications. Surveys from many of those who request the drug but don't take it say they feel comforted knowing that it's an option.

Some have warned that the laws might result in a decline of palliative care and hospice services as patients choose to die early instead of seeking such care, but this has not materialized. The availability of hospice and palliative care has expanded substantially in these states in recent years. And reports from Oregon show that nearly all the patients who used the state's Death with Dignity Act were using hospice care at the time of their deaths.

CHOOSING—AND CHOOSING AGAIN

As I've learned from my patients since the Washington State law took affect, having access to aid in dying doesn't necessarily make the choice straightforward. I have seen people who assumed they would choose physician-assisted death change their minds once they found themselves getting closer to dying. And I have seen people who were certain that physician-assisted death was wrong—not only for themselves but for others—until they were faced with their own terminal illness. Then they changed their minds entirely.

The lesson, I believe—for patients, their care providers, families, and others—is to keep an open heart and an open mind over time. In this way, we can help individuals find a way to die according to their most dearly held wishes and values. And there's no reason people should be afraid to change their minds about physician-assisted death as circumstances in their lives change.

I saw this lesson unfold in a most extraordinary way a few years ago with my friend and patient Charlotte Brooks. As I described in chapter 3, Charlotte was well versed in care of the dying. Her husband, Roger, benefited from hospice care when he was living and dying with pancreatic cancer. Also, Charlotte had been a nurse and strong advocate for improvements in long-term care. So when the Death with Dignity Act promoting physician-assisted death came before Washington voters in 2008, the community looked to Charlotte as an opinion leader. She had been a proponent of a similar ballot measure in 1991. Having seen too many patients linger in pain and emotional stress while terminally ill, the proposed law appealed to her as a compassionate choice.

But by 2008, Charlotte's perspective had changed with the world around her. The hospice movement was making great progress in addressing the needs of dying people, especially those with cancer. Also, Charlotte knew that if Roger had chosen assisted death when he was first diagnosed and given only six months to live—she might never have experienced the twenty-eight months they unexpectedly had together between his diagnosis and the time he died. She told others that she had learned life is precious to the end, that it's possible to alleviate a dying person's misery without ending life.

Charlotte did not foresee, however, that she would have cause to change her mind once again.

Sadly, in the summer of 2014, Charlotte discovered a prominent lump in her breast and was eventually diagnosed with advanced breast cancer. The doctors recommended treatment with surgery, radiation, or chemotherapy that might extend her life for several months, but it could not bring a cure. At age eighty-eight, Charlotte decided she would not seek treatment. She was already using a walker for balance and mobility, and her endurance was waning. She felt there was no point in medical intervention that would likely bring additional suffering. To her, the most important thing was to use the time she had to its best advantage, and that would require preserving her energy and maintaining a clear mind. So instead of treatment, Charlotte asked her doctors for a referral to hospice care, which had served Roger so well.

Charlotte envisioned that her death would be like Roger's, and that she would not need extra assistance to die peacefully. By late summer, however, Charlotte raised the idea of "death with dignity" with Denise LeFevre, a confidant and nursing colleague. Since Roger's death, Denise and Kyle Thomas, another colleague, had become a surrogate family to Charlotte, who had no children of her own. The three shared a love of nursing and education. Now Charlotte turned to them because she had begun to worry, Denise said.[16]

Their discussions about aid in dying were tentative at first. "She felt uncomfortable that she had changed her mind," Kyle explained, "but she said it was an evolution. When she spoke out against the Death with Dignity law in 2008, it was in the context of Roger's [recent] death."[17] She felt that if people cut their lives short too soon, they might miss the kind of meaningful experiences she and Roger had had—even in the throes of his illness. But now faced with her own death—at a different time, under different circumstances—she didn't feel the same way at all.

It wasn't the physical limitations of illness that bothered Charlotte so much. She had resources to hire caregivers she needed to meet her personal needs. But she placed a high value on thinking lucidly, expressing herself clearly, socializing, and contributing to her community. Following her diagnosis, she kept serving on committees in the large retirement community where she lived. And although retired, she still conversed regularly with colleagues at her workplace.

For Charlotte, an enjoyable life meant "being able to connect with people," Kyle said. She was a hub of social interaction in every community she belonged to. "She loved to have dinner with people, have them over for a meaningful conversation."

But as her illness progressed, she grew weaker. Finding energy for these activities grew harder and harder.

Soon Charlotte began wondering aloud about how her death would occur, Denise remembered. Would she become so incapacitated that she would no longer be able to eat? Would she develop pneumonia from weakness? What would be her actual cause of death? One day, she asked Denise if it was wrong to simply "skip" those last hours, days, and weeks. But before Denise could respond, Charlotte answered the question herself. No, it wasn't wrong.

So Charlotte told her hospice-team physician she was ready to file the papers needed to get the medication that would end her life. She asked me, as her primary care doctor, to serve as the "consulting physician"—the second doctor needed to verify that she met the provisions of the law.

Once Charlotte made her decision, she faced constant questioning from her doctors, caregivers, and friends, said Kyle. Over and over, people would ask her, "Are you sure?" And over and over, she told them, "Yes, I am sure."

Knowing that some friends might have moral or religious objections, Charlotte played her cards close to the chest. But among those she told, her favorite response was, "I wish you a peaceful journey."

Some of the toughest grilling came from professionals who regularly work with older people or the dying. A manager at the retirement community where she lived said (incorrectly) that "the law" did not allow such activity within the facility. A geriatrician said (again, incorrectly) that she would need to go to a hotel to take the medication that would aid in her dying. Hospice workers evaded logistical questions.

"Charlotte was furious," said Kyle. "She said, 'This is my home and you're telling me I cannot do what I am planning to do?' So she had to fight them, but it was the kind of challenge she thrived on." And, of course, Charlotte prevailed.

By December 2014, Charlotte was ready. She called her close friends to set the date.

"It was one of the strangest conversations I've ever had," Kyle remembered. "I never expected that somebody would one day ask me, 'Kyle, would it be okay with you if I die on Wednesday?' I felt speechless. . . . All I could say was, 'Huh?'"

And yet, Charlotte decided to have fun with her dear friend.

"She said, 'If it doesn't work for your schedule on Wednesday, then perhaps we can postpone it until Thursday or Friday.' And eventually it happened on Friday because that worked out best for everybody."

On the night before, Charlotte held a farewell party with six of her closest friends in the dining room at her retirement community. After dinner, they went to Charlotte's small apartment to share dessert and a celebratory bottle of wine.

"It was a lovely dinner," Kyle said. "The conversation was about Charlotte's legacy—her life and contribution to society." As the evening wore down, each guest kissed Charlotte on the cheek and said goodbye.

The next morning, Kyle and Denise arrived at Charlotte's apartment. Charlotte was in her bed, in her bathrobe. "We sat and talked again about her legacy," Kyle recalled. "Charlotte loved her iPad, so we Googled her name." The machine brought up historic photos and information about all that Charlotte had accomplished in her career and contributed to the field of nursing. "So we had a lively conversation about that."

Then Charlotte was ready. Denise mixed the medication into pear applesauce with fresh ginger that she had made especially for the occasion because the drug is known to taste bitter.

They handed the bowl to Charlotte. She ate all of it, and within minutes she told her friends that she felt sleepy. Kyle and Denise held her hand. Over the next five minutes, Charlotte's breathing grew slower and slower until if finally stopped.

"It was quite an emotional moment to see someone you love and appreciate fading away," said Kyle. "It was like a one-way journey, and we knew this was the last conversation we were going to have."

Denise said she thinks Charlotte would want us to know that she had a good death. "I think she would say that the only thing she missed was the last 'icky' part of dying. She enjoyed every bit of life, right up to the end, where she orchestrated the day, the setting, who was there, how it went. We could see in the last few days that it was becoming very difficult for her. She was ready."

As a former ICU nurse, Denise had seen many people die, but she said Charlotte's death was different. "She seemed so at peace and in control. She suffered minimally. . . . She was not afraid."

Denise added, "What we did that day was a gift to Charlotte, but it was also something very sacred, something that should only be done within the context of a loving relationship where you can feel sure that your intentions are pure and kind."

In their careers, both Denise and Kyle had examined end-of-life choices and the issue of assisted death from many perspectives—including its political and ethical implications. But participating in Charlotte's death seemed apart from all of this, they said. Charlotte had asked for their support to do something that mattered deeply, and they felt honored to help her. "Everything happened on her terms, exactly as she envisioned."

A CHOICE FOR THOSE DISABLED BUT NOT TERMINAL

As today's generation of middle-aged people considers planning for aging and eventual death, can experiences like Charlotte's be a model? The answer depends on the choices available to individuals and what they value. I believe boomers—especially those who take an activist approach—will be more likely to seek the kind of autonomy and comfort Charlotte achieved through the support of her friends, her caregivers, and her community's "death with dignity" law.

Physician-aided death is a complex issue. Many have strong feelings both in favor and against. It's anybody's guess whether the boomer generation, which powered so many revolutionary changes in the way we live, will also power revolutionary change in the way we die. I predict the boomers will. But whether they find the same solace experienced by Charlotte and her companions in dying may be determined by many factors—including their community's legal restrictions on physician-assisted death.

For those who don't meet the legal qualifications for physician-aided dying, or who live in places that don't allow it, choosing a humane self-activated death is difficult but not impossible. One common approach is to voluntarily stop eating and drinking—a legal choice that many physicians support.

That's the choice my close friend and patient John Cushman made a few years after Charlotte died. John was in his mideighties and traveling in another city when he experienced a sudden, massive stroke. I was not part of his initial care team when he returned by air ambulance to Seattle. But I soon visited him at the medical center, where he was about to receive state-of-the-art rehabilitation therapy.

I'll never forget John's expression when he saw me walk into his hospital room. Though partially paralyzed and unable to speak in a normal tone, he smiled for the first time in days according to his wife. I believe it was a smile of relief at seeing the doctor who had cared for him for nearly forty years, who had known him well before this catastrophic event.

John waited until the nurse looked away. Then, in voiceless speech, he mouthed these words three times for emphasis: "Get me out of here. Get me out of here. Get me out of here."

For weeks, John had been under the care of a very competent team of physicians and nurses. I consulted with his neurologists, who showed me his brain scans. I discussed his rehabilitation plans and potential for improvement with the hospital's head of rehabilitation medicine. They told me his mental abilities were fine, but given the damage the stroke had caused, there was little hope that he would regain much physical function. Still, his team had developed a plan that would allow him to return to his multilevel home, although he would be restricted to a single floor. Eventually, he might be able to move about safely in a wheelchair. But he would never walk again. He would sleep in a hospital bed. He would need personal assistance.

I already had an inkling of how John felt about this. His brother had suffered a similar stroke a few years earlier. John came to see me shortly after a visit with his brother, which he found emotionally devastating. He had described his brother's life as "miserable" and "tragic," something he could not imagine for himself. If the same thing ever happened to him, John said, he would rather be dead. And now here he was.

John had heard about Charlotte's death through a mutual friend. "I want to do what she did," he told me. He wanted me to help him die. But for me to assist John in getting medication to take his own life would be illegal. Unlike Charlotte, John was not terminally ill, just seriously disabled. And his stroke was relatively recent. He had experienced little if any recognizable recovery of function. His prognosis was grim, but he wasn't dying.

Still, I felt that John was making a legitimate, reasoned request based on his longing to end his anguish and suffering, and I felt that as his physician, I had an obligation to listen and respond in a way that would serve him best. Like many of my patients, John was a highly accomplished individual, capable of developing strong opinions that were well thought out. And he was fiercely independent. He was a take-charge person.

In the end, John and I chose another option—one that has always been available and has been chosen from time immemorial by people with health conditions that make living unacceptable to them. He decided that he would no longer eat or drink. He would also stop taking medications other than for comfort.

Once a patient makes this choice, the process usually takes a few days before dehydration causes death to occur. Although thirst and hunger may be uncomfortable at first, those feelings typically pass in a day or two and can be alleviated with sedatives.

I explained all of this to John and his wife. And then John, his wife, and I discussed it with their grown children, who appeared devastated at the prospect. Clearly, the family did not want to lose their beloved husband and father. But ultimately they seemed to understand that this needed to be his decision and they would try to respect his wishes. And after some consideration, John decided this was what he wanted to do. So we made arrangements for him to leave the hospital and return home, where he would have no food or liquids except as he might seek for comfort. He died five days later, peacefully and in the presence of his family.

My decision to help John in this situation was not made lightly. I don't know any physician for whom it would be. But after forty years of medical practice, I feel certain that health care needs to offer people a path beyond continuous intervention—especially when such treatment goes against the patient's deepest wishes.

I also believe it's my duty as a physician to respect a person's choices. Older individuals such as John, Charlotte, and Rolando have gained wisdom through their experience, observation, and reflection. Some call it "the wisdom of the elderly." This wisdom can be our teacher, providing lessons—both sad and profound—about life's meaning and worth.

For Charlotte, who had no remaining family, making the choice was difficult because she knew assisted death is irreversible—there's no turning back. For people like John and most others with family, the decisions and ultimate actions are much more complicated. Nearly always, and John's case is no exception, family members, especially children and spouses, object to the decision John made: "I want to stop eating and drinking, go to sleep, and just die." John's family loved their father and husband and did not want to live their lives without him. But ultimately, John knew all this and still made a conscious decision. And I believe that choice needed to be respected and honored. It's my duty to listen, to question, and ultimately to respond to my patient's decision. At the same time it's my duty to explain to those who are about to be bereaved, "It's okay. This is what John wants, and I hope that you can understand and accept this course he's chosen."

Most importantly, I believe such decisions must be rooted in the individual patient's wishes and values. I would only provide this kind of support for patients I know well and whose motives I understand. Death is sacred, mysterious, and irreversible; therefore, I would never want to risk miscalculating my patient's intent in seeking it as a peaceful relief from illness and suffering.

AND IN THE END . . .

By the time the baby-boom generation grows very old, science and medicine will have amassed tremendous knowledge about aging and death, thanks in large part to lessons learned from the experience of our parents' cohort, the Greatest Generation. Ideally, research conducted in huge populations of elderly people who died from strokes, cancer, heart disease, Alzheimer's disease, and more will help us to improve the way end-of-life care is designed and delivered. It will help us to approach death with some sense of comfort, knowing the following:

- We have the support we need to live and die in a way that aligns with our wishes and values.

- We have safeguards in place to ensure that decisions about our care will be made thoughtfully and ethically.
- We have made choices and communicated our decisions to our physicians, caregivers, relatives, and friends.
- We can revisit our choices at any time, allowing ourselves to change our minds as our circumstances and values change.

But in the end, it's the individual lives and deaths that the boomers will remember. We'll think of people like John Cushman, Charlotte Brooks, Rolando Perez, Evangeline Shuler, and others and recall the great lessons their living and dying taught us. We'll remember what made them happy, what caused them to suffer, and what seemed to relieve their suffering. And if we're wise, we'll take those lessons to heart as we prepare for our own individual endings. We will become resilient, "enlightened" agers—taking a proactive stance for own well-being; accepting the challenges inherent in aging; and building the mental, physical, and social reserves to live happily until the end.

For most of us, few stories will hold more meaning than the death of our own parents.

As I described in chapter 5, my father, Palmer Larson, faced many joys and struggles in his ninety-six years on this earth. In retirement, he enjoyed spending winters in the Arizona desert, welcoming his grandchildren into the world, and eventually settling in at the Rose Villa Retirement Community near Portland, Oregon.

But the years prior to his death were not easy ones. His mind had begun to slip—so much so that he eventually had to move into the community's health center and could no longer live with my mother. He struggled mightily with the loss of his mental capacity, referring to his confusion as his "curse." He suffered difficult behaviors, perhaps because of adverse drug effects. Through it all, however, he displayed a kind of strength, equanimity, and resilience that amazed my sister, Grethe Ann, and me. Each time he had a serious setback, we would encourage his health care team to evaluate him for hospice care. And not once—but two times—he was admitted to a hospice unit, only to "graduate" from it after his condition improved. We actually said, "Our dad failed hospice!"

Near the end, Dad had more difficulty with normal conversation but loved to listen. Occasionally, he was able to speak heart to heart with my sister, my mother, and me about matters that were very important in our family and his life. He always knew our spouses and his grandkids by name. He repeatedly expressed how much he loved our mother and how much he loved us, his "kids." In fact, he called himself "the richest man on earth."

He had a strong and abiding Christian faith that seemed to comfort him. He told me he was "ready to go to Jesus." Remarkably, he never lost his ability to pray. And even when he could remember nothing else, he was able to say the Lord's Prayer, our family's mealtime blessing, or a prayer he had learned in Norwegian as a boy.

One day in 2012, he unexpectedly developed intense pain through-out his body with no apparent cause. My family had decided together that we would not subject him to the confusion and stress of emergency medical care. Instead, we talked with his care providers to be sure that he had the medication he needed to stay as comfortable and pain free as possible. We knew his death was near.

Over the next four days, Grethe Ann, my mother, or I sat at his bedside, holding his hand. He was aware of our presence, but we didn't talk much. There was a closeness, a connection among us as the time passed in silence.

On the eve of his death, Dad stopped talking and fell into a deep sleep. We expected he would stop breathing soon. At one point, my sister left the room, emotionally drained. She returned about an hour later and stood next to Dad at his bedside. She smiled warmly and said to him, "Hi, Dad! How are you?" For the first time in hours, he opened his eyes and looked at all three of us.

"I'm fine," he said clearly and serenely before closing his eyes again. Those were his last words.

I realized at that moment that Dad could have given us no greater gift. After all his struggle, he had come to this place of peace. With his simple words, he was telling us just what we needed to hear: All is well. We can rest in death. We have nothing to fear.

UNTIL THEN

It's a message I try to keep in mind as I care for patients facing the ends of their lives. I also try to remember it as I contemplate my own inevitable ending. Like most of my boomer friends and relatives, I hope and expect to be around for a few more decades, even as I become increasingly aware of my mind and body aging.

To maximize my chances of living long and well, I intend to stay active. I'll keep riding my bike to the office as much as possible—including on rainy Seattle mornings. And even as I plan for retirement, I don't see myself retiring mentally, physically, socially, or spiritually. The breadth of my focus may narrow, but I anticipate I will always be seeking ways to add meaning and understanding to my life and the lives of those around me, especially my family. I hope my wife and I will get more time together to pursue both hobbies and volunteer work in our community. And I hope we will have more days to enjoy our children and our growing brood of grandkids.

I will heed the lessons I've accrued—those I learned from having had the privilege of being a physician and scientist, and those I learned from just living. I'll try to follow my own advice to be an enlightened, activist ager—that is, one who keeps learning and adapting to limitations that come with growing older. I'll seek only as much medical care as I need to live in accord with my goals. Like most people I've met, I don't want my life and well-being to be a burden to others. I will try to accept the things I cannot change with equanimity.

And when it comes time to die, I will be grateful to all my patients, colleagues, and friends—and especially to my beloved family—who have made my life well worth living.

ACKNOWLEDGMENTS

While it would be a fool's errand to try to thank all the people who have influenced the development of this book, I will attempt to call out those whose contributions are top of mind. First, I want to acknowledge Paul Beeson and Robert Petersdorf, who encouraged my nascent interest in aging and offered me their wise and unfailing support early in my career.

Because aging is multidimensional, interdisciplinary collaboration is key to advancing our understanding of it. This has been especially true in my work. So I wish to thank colleagues in the University of Washington (UW) Departments of Medicine, Psychiatry, Epidemiology, and Pathology who were stalwarts as we developed our research programs together. In addition to Burton Reifler, this includes Bud Kukull, George Martin, Bill Hazzard, and the University of British Columbia's Lynn Beattie—all of whom provided their unfailing encouragement and partnership early in my career. Later on, this circle widened to include Paul Crane, Ed Wagner, Gil Omenn, Tom Montine, and other great supporters at Group Health Research Institute (GHRI) and the UW, who have contributed immensely to our work.

I also want to acknowledge the National Institute on Aging's (NIA's) fabulous project officers who have been supportive over many years. The ACT study would not have been possible without NIA's funding of our research proposals over so many years.

And of course a huge measure of credit goes to our Alzheimer's Disease Patient Registry/Adult Changes in Thought (ADPR/ACT) project teams at UW and GHRI for their ceaseless dedication to developing and nurturing our most precious resource—our population of thousands of ACT volunteers who have been part of the study, many for more than thirty years. Thanks to study leaders Meredith Pfanschmidt, Sheila O'Connell, and Darlene White, all recently retired after decades of service. And thanks to the many other staff members who worked so tirelessly to advance our research. Getting to know our ACT participants has been a labor of love for all of us.

Appreciation also goes to the Robert Wood Johnson Foundation for supporting the development of this book through a grant to the Princeton Fund. In addition, we received support from the Group Health Foundation's Geriatric Research Fund and the UW Foundation, for which we are grateful.

Thanks also to Group Health leaders, and especially Scott Armstrong, for the opportunity he provided for me to have sabbatical at Cambridge University and its Institute for Public Health Science in 2014. While there, Carol Brayne and her group graciously provided space and support for me as I began writing the book. It was a special time that my wife Teresa and I will treasure forever.

I also thank my colleagues at GHRI for all they've contributed over the years and for allowing me the time away at Cambridge. Thanks to my assistant Rita Weikal, who has helped keep me organized. And thanks, of course, to my coauthor, Joan DeClaire, a talented writer who has also been a great colleague and friend to me—especially as we have collaborated on this book.

And finally, I want to express my appreciation to my patients and their families. I have learned so much from knowing and caring for them throughout the years. Being part of their lives is a privilege that I treasure. Likewise, we have gained tremendous insight from the ACT study participants and their relatives whose participation has been critical to advancing knowledge that is benefiting so many.

NOTES

INTRODUCTION

1. Wan He and Mark N. Muenchrath, "90+ in the United States: 2006–2008," U.S. Census Bureau, American Community Survey Reports ACS-17, November 2011, 2.

1. WELCOME TO THE AGE OF ENLIGHTENMENT

1. Eric B. Larson et al., "Exercise Is Associated with Reduced Risk for Incident Dementia among Persons 65 Years of Age and Older," *Annals of Internal Medicine* 144 (2006): 73–81.

2. Lynn Chalmers, phone interview with authors, Seattle, March 18, 2015.

3. Wan He and Mark N. Muenchrath, "90+ in the United States: 2006–2008." U.S. Census Bureau, American Community Survey Reports ACS-17, November 2011, 2.

4. Ibid.

5. Ibid., 16.

6. Marcus Aquino (pseudonym), interview with authors, Seattle, March 9, 2015.

7. Heather P. Lacey, Dylan M. Smith, and Peter A. Ubel, "Hope I Die before I Get Old: Mispredicting Happiness across the Adult Lifespan," *Journal of Happiness Studies* 7 (2006): 167–82.

8. Eric B. Larson et al., "Adverse Drug Reactions Associated with Global Cognitive Impairment in Elderly Persons," *Annals of Internal Medicine* 107 (1987): 169–73.

9. Linda Teri, Rebecca G. Logsdon, and Susan M. McCurry, "Exercise Interventions for Dementia and Cognitive Impairment: The Seattle Protocols," *Journal of Nutrition, Health & Aging* 12, no. 6 (2008): 391–94.

10. Dariush Mozaffarian et al., "Executive Summary: Heart Disease and Stroke Statistics—2016 Update: A Report from the American Heart Association," *Circulation* 133 (2016): 447–54.

11. Rebecca Hughes, "ACT Study: Long-Running Study of Aging Examines Changes in Group Health Patients over Time," Group Health Research Institute, July 1, 2015, https://www.grouphealthresearch.org/our-research/research-areas/aging-geriatrics/act-study-long-running-study-aging-examines-changes-group-health-patients-over-time/.

12. Joe Feldman and Lena Feldman (pseudonyms), interview with authors, Seattle, June 16, 2016.

13. Joshua Sonnen et al., "Neuropathology in the Adult Changes in Thought Study: A Review," *Journal of Alzheimer's Disease* 18 (2009): 703–11.

2. PROACTIVITY

1. Lynn Chalmers, phone interview with authors, Seattle, March 18, 2015.

2. "History," OurBodiesOurselves.org, http://www.ourbodiesourselves.org/history/.

3. Jennifer M. Ortman, Victoria A. Velkoff, and Howard Hogan, "An Aging Nation: The Older Population in the United States," U.S. Census Bureau, Current Population Reports P25-1140, May 2014, 1.

4. Linda Babcock, phone interview with authors, Seattle, April 8, 2015.

5. Dana E. King et al., "The Status of Baby Boomers' Health in the United States: The Healthiest Generation?," *JAMA Internal Medicine* 173, no. 5 (2013): 385–86.

6. Elizabeth M. Badley et al., "Benefits Gained, Benefits Lost: Comparing Baby Boomers to Other Generations in a Longitudinal Cohort Study of Self-Rated Health," *Milbank Quarterly* 93, no. 1 (2015): 40–72.

7. National Center for Health Statistics, *Health, United States, 2015: With Special Feature on Racial and Ethnic Health Disparities* (Hyattsville, MD: National Center for Health Statistics, 2016), 210.

8. Barbara Bronson Gray, "Boomers' Health Fails to Measure up to Parents'," *HealthDay News*, February 4, 2013, https://consumer.healthday.com/senior-citizen-information-31/age-health-news-7/boomers-health-fails-to-measure-up-to-parents-673170.html.

9. Tara Parker-Pope, "Overtreatment Is Taking a Harmful Toll," *New York Times*, August 27, 2012, http://well.blogs.nytimes.com/2012/08/27/over-treatment-is-taking-a-harmful-toll/?_r=0.

10. Lisa Chedekel, "Overdiagnosis: Bad for You, Good for Business; SPH Bicknell Lecturer Says Too Much Treatment Makes People Sick," *Boston University Today*, October 26, 2011, http://www.bu.edu/today/2011/medical-over-diagnosis-bad-for-you-good-for-business/.

11. Ibid.

12. H. Gilbert Welch et al., "Breast-Cancer Tumor Size, Overdiagnosis, and Mammography Screening Effectiveness," *New England Journal of Medicine* 375, no. 15 (2016): 1438–47.

13. H. Gilbert Welch, "When Screening Is Bad for a Woman's Health," *Los Angeles Times*, July 19, 2015.

14. Kevin C. Oeffinger et al., "Breast Cancer Screening for Women at Average Risk: 2015 Guideline Update from the American Cancer Society," *JAMA* 314, no. 15 (2015): 1599–1614.

15. U.S. Preventive Services Task Force, "Final Update Summary: Breast Cancer: Screening," http://www.uspreventiveservicestaskforce.org/Page/Document/UpdateSummaryFinal/breast-cancer-screening1.

16. Jeffrey Jarvik et al., "The Longitudinal Assessment of Imaging and Disability of the Back (LAIDBack) Study: Baseline Data," *Spine* 26 (2001): 1158–66.

17. National Public Radio, "Is Preventive Medicine Actually Overtreatment?," *Science Friday*, February 11, 2011, http://www.npr.org/2011/02/11/133686016/Is-Preventive-Medicine-Actually-Overtreatment.

18. John N. Mafi et al., "Worsening Trends in the Management and Treatment of Back Pain," *JAMA Internal Medicine* 173, no. 17 (2013): 1573–81.

19. Steven J. Stack, "A Call to Action: Physicians Must Turn the Tide of the Opioid Epidemic," *AMA Wire*, February 17, 2016. http://www.ama-assn.org/ama/ama-wire/post/call-action-physicians-must-turn-tide-of-opioid-epidemic.

20. Michael Von Korff and Gary Franklin, "Responding to America's Iatrogenic Epidemic of Prescription Opioid Addiction and Overdose," *Medical Care* 54, no. 5 (2016): 426–29.

21. Stack, "Call to Action."

22. Writing Group for the Women's Health Initiative Investigators, "Risks and Benefits of Estrogen Plus Progestin in Healthy Postmenopausal Women: Principal Results from the Women's Health Initiative Randomized Controlled Trial," *JAMA* 288, no. 3 (2002): 321–33.

23. Chedekel, "Overdiagnosis."

24. Mike Evans, "23 and 1/2 Hours: What Is the Single Best Thing I Can Do for My Health?," Evans Health Lab, http://www.evanshealthlab.com/23-and-12-hours/.

25. Kirk Williamson, phone interview with authors, Seattle, June 29, 2016.

26. David Arterburn, Emily O. Westbrook, and Clarissa Hsu, "Case Study: The Shared Decision Making Story at Group Health," in *Shared Decision Making in Health Care: Achieving Evidence-Based Patient Choice*, 3rd ed., ed. Glyn Elwyn, Adrian Edwards, and Rachel Thompson, 190–96 (New York City: Oxford University Press, 2016).

27. Jaime King and Benjamin Moulton, "Group Health's Participation in a Shared Decision-Making Demonstration Yielded Lessons, Such as Role of Culture Change," *Health Affairs* 32, no. 2 (2013): 294–302.

28. Annette M. O'Connor et al., "Decision Aids for People Facing Health Treatment or Screening Decisions," *Cochrane Database of Systematic Reviews*, no. 1 (2003).

29. David Arterburn et al., "Introducing Decision Aids at Group Health Was Linked to Sharply Lower Hip and Knee Surgery Rates and Costs," *Health Affairs* 31, no. 9 (2012): 2094–2104.

30. Melissa Parson and Rebecca Hughes, "Three (Amazing) Group Health Patients Tell Stories of Participating in Our Research," Group Health Research Institute, April 22, 2016, https://www.grouphealthresearch.org/news-and-events/blog/2016/april/watch-our-new-video-group-health-research-made-real/.

31. Wendy Townsend, interview with authors, Seattle, June 2, 2016.

3. ACCEPTANCE

1. Meredith Pfanschmidt, interview with authors, Seattle, April 29, 2015.

2. Milena Nikolova and Carol Graham, "Employment, Late-Life Work, Retirement, and Well-Being in Europe and the United States," *IZA Journal of European Labor Studies* 3, no. 5 (2014): 1–30.

3. Fred Dews, "This Happiness and Age Chart Will Leave You with a Smile (Literally)," Brookings Institute, March 28, 2014, https://www.brookings.edu/blog/brookings-now/2014/03/28/this-happiness-age-chart-will-leave-you-with-a-smile-literally/.

4. Hannes Schwandt, "Unmet Aspirations as an Explanation for the Age U-Shape in Wellbeing," *Journal of Economic Behavior and Organization* 122 (2016): 75–87.

5. Hannes Schwandt, "Why So Many of Us Experience a Mid-Life Crisis," *Harvard Business Review*, April 20, 2015.

6. Elizabeth Gilbert, "The Most Strangely Reassuring Advice I Ever Received," ElizabethGilbert.com, October 8, 2014, http://www.elizabethgilbert.com/the-most-strangely-reassuring-advice-i-ever-received-long-ago-when-i-was-in-m/.

7. Laura L. Carstensen, "The Influence of a Sense of Time on Human Development," *Science* 312 (2006): 1913–15.

8. Daniel Goleman, "Erikson, in His Own Old Age, Expands His View of Life," *New York Times*, June 14, 1988.

9. Bob Zufall, phone interview with authors, Seattle, June 25, 2015.

10. Stephen G. Post, "Altruism, Happiness, and Health: It's Good to Be Good," *International Journal of Behavioral Medicine* 12 (2005): 66–77.

11. Ray Moynihan and Alan Cassels, *Selling Sickness: How the World's Biggest Pharmaceutical Companies Are Turning Us All into Patients* (New York: Nation Books, 2005).

12. Dennis McCullough, *My Mother, Your Mother: Embracing "Slow Medicine," the Compassionate Approach to Caring for Your Aging Loved Ones* (New York: HarperCollins, 2008).

13. Dennis McCullough, "Slow Medicine," *Dartmouth Medicine*, Spring 2008.

14. John W. Rowe and Robert L. Kahn, "Successful Aging," *Gerontologist* 37 (1997): 433–40.

4. BUILD YOUR RESERVES FOR RESILIENCE

1. James F. Fries, "Aging, Natural Death, and the Compression of Morbidity, 1980," *Bulletin of the World Health Organization* 80, no. 3 (2002): 245–50.

2. James F. Fries, Bonnie Bruce, and Eliza Chakravarty, "Compression of Morbidity 1980–2011: A Focused Review of Paradigms and Progress," *Journal of Aging Research* (2011): article ID 261702, https://www.hindawi.com/journals/jar/2011/261702/ref/.

3. Pseudonym for composite sources interviewed by authors, June 2016.

4. Family member of Ben Stevenson (pseudonym), interview with authors, Seattle, April 29, 2016.

5. BUILDING YOUR MENTAL RESERVES

1. Kirk Erickson et al., "Exercise Training Increases Size of Hippocampus and Improves Memory," *Proceedings of the National Academy of Sciences of the USA* 108 (2011): 3017–22.

2. Allen Roses, "On the Discovery of the Genetic Association of Apolipoprotein E Genotypes and Common Late-Onset Alzheimer Disease," *Journal of Alzheimer's Disease* 9, no. 3 (2006): S361–66.

3. George S. Zubenko et al., "Family Study of Platelet Membrane Fluidity in Alzheimer's Disease," *Science* 238 (1987): 539–42.

4. Catharine L. Joachim, Hiroshi Mori, and Dennis J. Selkoe, "Amyloid Beta-Protein Deposition in Tissues Other Than Brain in Alzheimer's Disease," *Nature* 341, no. 6239 (1989): 226–30.

5. Ingmar Skoog et al., "A Population-Based Study of Dementia in 85-Year-Olds," *New England Journal of Medicine* 328, no. 3 (1993): 153–58.

6. Alfredo Lim et al., "Clinico-neuropathological Correlation of Alzheimer's Disease in a Community-Based Case Series," *Journal of the American Geriatrics Society* 47, no. 5 (1999): 564–69.

7. G. Blessed, B. E. Tomlinson, and Martin Roth, "The Association between Quantitative Measures of Dementia and of Senile Change in the Cerebral Grey Matter of Elderly Subjects," *British Journal of Psychiatry*, no. 114 (1968): 797–811.

8. Victoria Moceri et al., "Using Census Data and Birth Certificates to Reconstruct the Early-Life Socioeconomic Environment and the Relation to the Development of Alzheimer's Disease," *Epidemiology* 12 (2001): 383–89.

9. Hsiu-Chih Lui et al., "Assessing Cognitive Abilities and Cementia in a Predominantly Illiterate Population of Older Individuals in Kinmen," *Psychological Medicine*, no. 24 (1994): 763–70.

10. Sherry L. Willis et al., "Long-Term Effects of Cognitive Training on Everyday Functional Outcomes in Older Adults," *JAMA* 296, no. 23 (2006): 2805–14.

11. Eric B. Larson and Robert A. Bruce, "Exercise and Aging," *Annals of Internal Medicine* 105 (1986): 783–85.

12. Laura Fratiglioni, Stephanie Paillard-Borg, and Bengt Winblad, "An Active and Socially Integrated Lifestyle in Late Life Might Protect against Dementia," *Lancet Neurology* 3, no. 6 (2004): 343–53.

13. Joe Verghese et al., "Leisure Activities and the Risk of Dementia in the Elderly," *New England Journal of Medicine* 348, no. 25 (2003): 2508–16.

14. Eric B. Larson et al., "Exercise Is Associated with Reduced Risk for Incident Dementia among Persons 65 Years of Age and Older," *Annals of Internal Medicine* 144 (2006): 73–81.

15. Nicola Lautenschlager et al., "Effect of Physical Activity on Cognitive Function in Older Adults at Risk for Alzheimer Disease: A Randomized Trial," *JAMA* 300, no. 9 (2008): 1027–37.

16. Linda Teri et al., "Exercise Plus Behavioral Management in Patients with Alzheimer Disease: A Randomized Controlled Trial," *JAMA* 290, no. 15 (2003): 2015–22.

17. Anahad O'Connor, "Exercise and Setting Ease Alzheimer's Effects," *New York Times*, November 4, 2003.

18. Shelly L. Gray et al., "Cumulative Use of Strong Anticholinergic Medications and Incident Dementia," *JAMA Internal Medicine* 175, no. 3 (2015): 401–7.

19. Paul K. Crane et al., "Glucose Levels and Risk of Dementia," *New England Journal of Medicine* 369, no. 6 (2013): 540–48.

6. BUILDING YOUR PHYSICAL RESERVES

1. Fuzhong Li et al., "Tai Chi and Fall Reductions in Older Adults: A Randomized Controlled Trial," *Journal of Gerontology: Medical Sciences* 60, no. 2 (2005): 187–94; Alexander Voukelatos et al., "A Randomized, Controlled Trial of Tai Chi for the Prevention of Falls: The Central Sydney Tai Chi Trial," *Journal of the American Geriatrics Society* 55 (2007): 1185–91; Steven L. Wolf et al., "Reducing Frailty and Falls in Older Persons: An Investigation of Tai Chi and Computerized Balance Training," *Journal of the American Geriatrics Society* 44, no. 5 (1996): 489–97.

2. Thomas D. Koepsell et al., "Footwear Style and Risk of Falls in Older Adults," *Journal of the American Geriatrics Society* 52, no. 9 (2004): 1495–1501.

3. Anita K. Wagner et al., "Benzodiazepine Use and Hip Fractures in the Elderly: Who Is at Greatest Risk?," *Archives of Internal Medicine* 164, no. 14 (2004): 1567–72.

4. Maria A. Fiatarone et al., "High-Intensity Strength Training in Nonagenarians: Effects on Skeletal Muscle," *JAMA* 263, no. 22 (1990): 3029–34.

5. Karen J. Sherman et al., "Comparing Yoga, Exercise, and a Self-Care Book for Chronic Low Back Pain: A Randomized, Controlled Trial," *Annals of Internal Medicine* 143 (2005): 849–56.

6. Daniel C. Cherkin et al., "A Comparison of the Effects of 2 Types of Massage and Usual Care on Chronic Low Back Pain: A Randomized, Controlled Trial," *Annals of Internal Medicine* 155 (2011): 1–9.

7. Daniel C. Cherkin et al., "A Randomized Trial Comparing Acupuncture, Simulated Acupuncture, and Usual Care for Chronic Low Back Pain," *Archives of Internal Medicine* 169, no. 9 (2009): 858–66.

8. Daniel C. Cherkin et al., "Effect of Mindfulness-Based Stress Reduction vs. Cognitive Behavioral Therapy or Usual Care on Back Pain and Functional Limitations in Adults with Chronic Low Back Pain: A Randomized Clinical Trial," *JAMA* 315, no. 12 (2016): 1240–49.

9. SPRINT Research Group, "A Randomized Trial of Intensive versus Standard Blood-Pressure Control," *New England Journal of Medicine* 373 (2015): 2103–16.

10. Tobacco Control Research Branch of the National Cancer Institute, "The Rewards of Quitting," SmokeFree.gov, https://smokefree.gov/rewards-of-quitting.

11. U.S. Department of Health and Human Services, *The Health Consequences of Smoking—50 Years of Progress: A Report of the Surgeon General* (Atlanta: U.S. Department of Health and Human Services, Centers for Disease Control and Prevention, National Center for Chronic Disease Prevention and Health Promotion, Office on Smoking and Health, 2014).

12. Michael C. Fiore et al., *Treating Tobacco Use and Dependence: 2008 Update*, Clinical Practice Guideline (Rockville, MD: U.S. Department of Health and Human Services, Public Health Service, Agency for Healthcare Research and Quality, 2008).

13. Ulf Ekelund et al. for the Lancet Physical Activity Series 2 Executive Committee and the Lancet Sedentary Behaviour Working Group, "Does Physical Activity Attenuate, or Even Eliminate, the Detrimental Association of Sitting Time with Mortality? A Harmonised Meta-analysis of Data from More Than 1 Million Men and Women," *Lancet* 388, no. 10051 (2016): 1302–10.

14. Douglas Martin, "Robert A. Bruce Is Dead at 87; Pioneer of Cardiac Stress Test," *New York Times*, February 14, 2004.

15. Eleanor H. Bruce et al., "Comparison of Active Participants and Dropouts in CAPRI Cardiopulmonary Rehabilitation Programs," *American Journal of Cardiology* 37, no. 1 (1976): 53–60.

16. Eric B. Larson et al., "Exercise Is Associated with Reduced Risk for Incident Dementia among Persons 65 Years of Age and Older," *Annals of Internal Medicine* 144, no. 2 (2006): 73–81.

17. Ekelund et al., "Does Physical Activity Attenuate, or Even Eliminate, the Detrimental Association of Sitting Time with Mortality?"

18. Gerald Alexander, "Standing up for My Health," Group Health Research Institute, April 8, 2015, https://www.grouphealthresearch.org/news-and-events/blog/2015/04/standing-my-health.

19.   Dori E. Rosenberg et al., "The Feasibility of Reducing Sitting Time in Overweight and Obese Older Adults," *Health Education and Behavior* 42, no. 5 (2015): 669–76.

20.   Ekelund et al., "Does Physical Activity Attenuate."

21.   Haroon Saddique, "One Hour of Activity Needed to Offset Harmful Effects of Sitting at a Desk," *Guardian*, July 27, 2016.

22.   National Heart, Lung, and Blood Institute, "Description of the DASH Eating Plan," https://www.nhlbi.nih.gov/health/health-topics/topics/dash.

23.   Katherine Harmon, "Addicted to Fat: Overeating May Alter the Brain as Much as Hard Drugs," *Scientific American*, March 28, 2010.

24.   Herbert Benson, *The Relaxation Response* (New York: HarperCollins, 1975).

25.   Asfandyar Khan Niazi and Shaharyar Khan Niazi, "Mindfulness-Based Stress Reduction: A Non-pharmacological Approach for Chronic Illnesses," *North American Journal of Medical Sciences* 3, no. 1 (2011): 20–23.

26.   National Center for Complementary and Integrative Health, "Use of Complementary Health Approaches in the United States: National Health Interview Survey," https://nccih.nih.gov/research/statistics/NHIS/2012/mind-body/yoga.

27.   National Institute on Deafness and Other Communication Disorders, "Age-Related Hearing Loss," https://www.nidcd.nih.gov/sites/default/files/Documents/health/hearing/AgeRelatedHearingLoss_0.pdf.

28.   Marcos V. Goycoolea et al., "Effect of Life in Industrialized Societies on Hearing in Natives of Easter Island," *Laryngoscope* 96 (1986): 1391–96.

7. BUILDING YOUR SOCIAL RESERVES

1.   NIH Senior Health, "Long-Term Care: Frequently Asked Questions," http://nihseniorhealth.gov/longtermcare/faq/faq6.html.

2.   Barbara Perez (pseudonym), interview with authors, Seattle, May 12, 2016.

3.   Rebecca Perez (pseudonym), interview with authors, Seattle, May 12, 2016.

4.   Joe Feldman (pseudonym), interview with authors, Seattle, June 16, 2016.

5.   Genworth Financial, "Compare Long Term Care Costs across the United States," https://www.genworth.com/about-us/industry-expertise/cost-of-care.html.

6.   AARP, "Fact Sheet: Cohousing for Older Adults," http://www.aarp.org/home-garden/housing/info-03-2010/fs175.html.

7. Sheila Hoffman, interview with authors, Seattle, August 10, 2016.

8. Spencer Beard, interview with authors, Seattle, August 10, 2016.

9. Katherine F. Burn et al., "The Role of Grandparenting in Post-menopausal Women's Cognitive Health: Results from the Women's Healthy Aging Project (WHAP)," *Menopause* 21 (2014): 1069–74.

10. Jeff Goldsmith, *The Long Baby Boom: An Optimistic Vision for a Graying Generation* (Baltimore: Johns Hopkins University Press, 2008), 86.

11. Melissa Brown et al., "Working in Retirement: A 21st Century Phenomenon," Sloan Center on Aging and Work and the Families and Work Institute, July 2010, 1.

12. Insured Retirement Institute, "Boomer Expectations for Retirement 2016," http://www.irionline.org/resources/resources-detail-view/boomer-2016.

13. Goldsmith, *Long Baby Boom*, xiii–xiv.

14. Ibid., 51.

15. Milena Nikolova and Carol Graham, "Employment, Late-Life Work, Retirement, and Well-Being in Europe and the United States," *IZA Journal of European Labor Studies* 3, no. 5 (2014): 5.

16. Carol Graham and Milena Nikolova, "Why Aging and Working Makes Us Happy in 4 Charts," *Brookings*, March 28, 2014.

17. Joan K. Morris, Derek G. Cook, and A. Gerald Shaper, "Loss of Employment and Mortality," *BMJ* 308, no. 6937 (1994): 1135–39.

18. Tara Bahrampour, "This Is Your Brain on Retirement—Not Nearly as Sharp, Studies Are Finding," *Washington Post*, October 29, 2015.

19. Ursula M. Staudinger et al., "A Global View on the Effects of Work on Health in Later Life," *Gerontologist* 56, no. S2 (2016): 281–92; Esteban Calvo, Natalia Sarkisian, and Christopher R. Tamborini, "Causal Effects of Retirement Timing on Subjective Physical and Emotional Health," *Journals of Gerontology Series B: Psychological Sciences and Social Sciences* 68, no. 1 (2013): 73–84.

20. Susann Rohwedder and Robert J. Willis, "Mental Retirement," *Journal of Economic Perspectives: A Journal of the American Economic Association* 24, no. 1 (2010): 119–38.

21. Martina Celidoni, Chiara Dal Bianco, and Guglielmo Weber, "Early Retirement and Cognitive Decline: A Longitudinal Analysis Using SHARE Data," "Marco Fanno" Working Papers 174, Department of Economics and Management, University of Padua, December 2013.

22. Wendy Townsend, interview with authors, Seattle, June 2, 2016.

8. CHOOSE YOUR OWN ENDING

1. Rebecca Perez (pseudonym), interview with authors, Seattle, May 12, 2016.

2. Barbara Perez (pseudonym), Interview with authors, Seattle, May 12, 2016.

3. Philip A. Pizzo and David M. Walker, "Should We Practice What We Profess? Care near the End of Life," *New England Journal of Medicine* 372, no. 7 (2015): 595–98.

4. Joan M. Teno et al., "Change in End-of-Life Care for Medicare Beneficiaries: Site of Death, Place of Care, and Health Care Transitions in 2000, 2005, and 2009," *JAMA* 309, no. 5 (2013): 470–77.

5. Emily A. Meier et al., "Defining a Good Death (Successful Dying): Literature Review and a Call for Research and Public Dialogue," *American Journal of Geriatric Psychiatry* 24, no 4 (2016): 261–71.

6. Deborah Netburn, "What Does It Mean to Have a 'Good Death'?," *Los Angeles Times*, April 1, 2016.

7. Pseudonym for composite sources interviewed with authors, June 2016.

8. Maria J. Silveira, Wyndy Wiitala, and John Piette, "Advance Directive Completion by Elderly Americans: A Decade of Change," *Journal of the American Geriatrics Society* 62, no. 4 (2014): 706–10.

9. Dana Meyers (pseudonym), phone interview with authors, Seattle, May 27, 2016.

10. Institute of Medicine, *Dying in America: Improving Quality and Honoring Individual Preferences near the End of Life* (Washington, DC: National Academies Press, 2015).

11. Pizzo and Walker, "Should We Practice What We Profess?"

12. PerryUndem Research/Communication, "Physicians' Views toward Advance Care Planning and End-of-Life Care Conversations: Findings from a National Survey among Physicians Who Regularly Treat Patients 65 and Older," Cambia Health Foundation, April 2016.

13. Elisabeth Kubler-Ross, *On Death and Dying* (New York: Macmillan, 1969).

14. Jennifer S. Temel et al., "Early Palliative Care for Patients with Metastatic Non-small-cell Lung Cancer," *New England Journal of Medicine* 363, no. 8 (2010): 733–42.

15. Lynn Chalmers, phone interview with authors, Seattle, March 18, 2015.

16. Denise LeFevre (pseudonym), personal correspondence with authors, July 15–16, 2016.

17. Kyle Thomas (pseudonym), interview with authors, Seattle, May 13, 2015.

BIBLIOGRAPHY

AARP. "Fact Sheet: Cohousing for Older Adults." http://www.aarp.org/home-garden/housing/info-03-2010/fs175.html.

Arterburn, David, Emily O. Westbrook, and Clarissa Hsu. "Case Study: The Shared Decision Making Story at Group Health." In *Shared Decision Making in Health Care: Achieving Evidence-Based Patient Choice*, 3rd ed., edited by Glyn Elwyn, Adrian Edwards, and Rachel Thompson, 190–96. New York City: Oxford University Press, 2016.

Arterburn, David, et al. "Introducing Decision Aids at Group Health Was Linked to Sharply Lower Hip and Knee Surgery Rates and Costs." *Health Affairs* 31, no. 9 (2012): 2094–2104.

Badley, Elizabeth M., et al. "Benefits Gained, Benefits Lost: Comparing Baby Boomers to Other Generations in a Longitudinal Cohort Study of Self-Rated Health." *Milbank Quarterly* 93, no. 1 (2015): 40–72.

Bahrampour, Tara. "This Is Your Brain on Retirement—Not Nearly as Sharp, Studies Are Binding," *Washington Post*, October 29, 2015.

Benson, Herbert. *The Relaxation Response.* New York: HarperCollins, 1975.

Blessed, G., B. E. Tomlinson, and Martin Roth. "The Association between Quantitative Measures of Dementia and of Senile Change in the Cerebral Grey Matter of Elderly Subjects." *British Journal of Psychiatry*, 114 (1968): 797–811.

Brown, Melissa, et al. "Working in Retirement: A 21st Century Phenomenon." Sloan Center on Aging and Work and the Families and Work Institute, July 2010, 1.

Bruce, Eleanor H., et al. "Comparison of Active Participants and Dropouts in CAPRI Cardiopulmonary Rehabilitation Programs." *American Journal of Cardiology* 37, no. 1 (1976): 53–60.

Burn, Katherine F., et al. "The Role of Grandparenting in Post-menopausal Women's Cognitive Health: Results from the Women's Healthy Aging Project (WHAP)." *Menopause* 21 (2014): 1069–74.

Calvo, Esteban, Natalia Sarkisian, and Christopher R. Tamborini. "Causal Effects of Retirement Timing on Subjective Physical and Emotional Health." *Journals of Gerontology Series B: Psychological Sciences and Social Sciences* 68, no. 1 (2013): 73–84.

Carstensen, Laura. L. "The Influence of a Sense of Time on Human Development." *Science* 312 (2006): 1913–15.

Celidoni, Martina, Chiara Dal Bianco, and Guglielmo Weber. "Early Retirement and Cognitive Decline: A Longitudinal Analysis Using SHARE Data." "Marco Fanno" Working Papers 174, Department of Economics and Management, University of Padua, December 2013.

Chedekel, Lisa. "Overdiagnosis: Bad for You, Good for Business; SPH Bicknell Lecturer Says Too Much Treatment Makes People Sick." *Boston University Today*, October 26, 2011. http://www.bu.edu/today/2011/medical-overdiagnosis-bad-for-you-good-for-business/.

Cherkin, Daniel C., et al. "A Comparison of the Effects of 2 Types of Massage and Usual Care on Chronic Low Back Pain: A Randomized, Controlled Trial." *Annals of Internal Medicine* 155 (2011): 1–9.

———. "Effect of mindfulness-based stress reduction vs. cognitive behavioral therapy or usual care on back pain and functional limitations in adults with chronic low back pain: a randomized clinical trial." *JAMA* 315, no. 12 (2016): 1240–49.

———. "A Randomized Trial Comparing Acupuncture, Simulated Acupuncture, and Usual Care for Chronic Low Back Pain." *Archives of Internal Medicine* 169, no. 9 (2009): 858–66.

Crane, Paul K., et al. "Glucose Levels and Risk of Dementia." *New England Journal of Medicine* 369, no. 6 (2013): 540–48.

Dews, Fred. "This Happiness and Age Chart Will Leave You with a Smile (Literally)." Brookings Institute, March 28, 2014. https://www.brookings.edu/blog/brookings-now/2014/03/28/this-happiness-age-chart-will-leave-you-with-a-smile-literally/.

Dominantly Inherited Alzheimer Network. "DIAN Observational Study." http://www.dian-info.org.

Ekelund, Ulf, et al., for the Lancet Physical Activity Series 2 Executive Committee and the Lancet Sedentary Behaviour Working Group. "Does Physical Activity Attenuate, or Even Eliminate, the Detrimental Association of Sitting Time with Mortality? A Harmonised Meta-analysis of Data from More Than 1 Million Men and Women." *Lancet* 388, no. 10051 (2016): 1302–10.

Erickson, Kirk, et al. "Exercise Training Increases Size of Hippocampus and Improves Memory." *Proceedings of the National Academy of Sciences of the USA* 108 (2011): 3017–22.

Evans, Mike. "23 and a Half Hours: What Is the Single Best Thing I Can Do for My Health?" Evans Health Lab. http://www.evanshealthlab.com/23-and-12-hours/.

Fiatarone, Maria A., et al. "High-Intensity Strength Training in Nonagenarians: Effects on Skeletal Muscle." *JAMA* 263, no. 22 (1990): 3029–34.

Fiore, Michael C., et al. *Treating Tobacco Use and Dependence: 2008 Update.* Clinical Practice Guideline. Rockville, MD: U.S. Department of Health and Human Services, Public Health Service, Agency for Healthcare Research and Quality, 2008.

Fratiglioni, Laura, Stephanie Paillard-Borg, and Bengt Winblad. "An Active and Socially Integrated Lifestyle in Late Life Might Protect against Dementia." *Lancet Neurology* 3, no. 6, (2004): 343–53.

Fries, James F. "Aging, Natural Death, and the Compression of Morbidity, 1980." *Bulletin of the World Health Organization* 80, no.3 (2002): 245–50.

Fries, James F., Bonnie Bruce, and Eliza Chakravarty. "Compression of Morbidity 1980–2011: A Focused Review of Paradigms and Progress." *Journal of Aging Research* (2011): article ID 261702. https://www.hindawi.com/journals/jar/2011/261702/ref/.

Genworth Financial. "Compare Long Term Care Costs across the United States." https://www.genworth.com/about-us/industry-expertise/cost-of-care.html.

Gilbert, Elizabeth. "The Most Strangely Reassuring Advice I Ever Received." ElizabethGilbert.com, October 8, 2014. http://www.elizabethgilbert.com/the-most-strangely-reassuring-advice-i-ever-received-long-ago-when-i-was-in-m/.

Goldsmith, Jeff. *The Long Baby Boom: An Optimistic Vision for a Graying Generation.* Baltimore: Johns Hopkins University Press, 2008.

Goleman, Daniel. "Erikson, in His Own Old Age, Expands His View of Life." *New York Times*, June 14, 1988.

Goycoolea, Marcos V., et al. "Effect of Life in Industrialized Societies on Hearing in Natives of Easter Island." *Laryngoscope* 96 (1986): 1391–96.

Graham, Carol, and Milena Nikolova. "Why Aging and Working Makes Us Happy in 4 Charts." *Brookings*, March 28, 2014.

Gray, Barbara Bronson. "Boomers' Health Fails to Measure up to Parents." *HealthDay News*, February 4, 2013. https://consumer.healthday.com/senior-citizen-information-31/age-health-news-7/boomers-health-fails-to-measure-up-to-parents-673170.html.

Gray, Shelly L., et al. "Cumulative Use of Strong Anticholinergic Medications and Incident Dementia." *JAMA Internal Medicine* 175, no. 3 (2015): 401–7.

Group Health Research Institute. "Standing up for my health." Grouphealthresearch.org. https://www.grouphealthresearch.org/news-and-events/blog/2015/04/standing-my-health (accessed September 2, 2016).

Harmon, Katherine. "Addicted to Fat: Overeating May Alter the Brain as Much as Hard Drugs." *Scientific American*, March 28, 2010.

He, Wan, and Mark N. Muenchrath. "90+ in the United States: 2006–2008." U.S. Census Bureau, American Community Survey Reports ACS-17, November 2011.

Hsiu-Chih Lui, et al. "Assessing Cognitive Abilities and Dementia in a Predominantly Illiterate Population of Older Individuals in Kinmen." *Psychological Medicine*, no. 24 (1994): 763–70.

Hughes, Rebecca. "ACT Study: Long-Running Study of Aging Examines Changes in Group Health Patients over Time." Group Health Research Institute, July 1, 2015. https://www.grouphealthresearch.org/our-research/research-areas/aging-geriatrics/act-study-long-running-study-aging-examines-changes-group-health-patients-over-time/.

Institute of Medicine. *Dying in America: Improving Quality and Honoring Individual Preferences near the End of Life.* Washington, DC: National Academies Press, 2015.

Insured Retirement Institute. "Boomer Expectations for Retirement 2016." http://www.irionline.org/resources/resources-detail-view/boomer-2016.

Jarvik, Jeffrey, et al. "The Longitudinal Assessment of Imaging and Disability of the Back (LAIDBack) Study: Baseline Data." *Spine* 26 (2001): 1158–66.

Joachim, Catharine L., Hiroshi Mori, and Dennis J. Selkoe. "Amyloid Beta-Protein Deposition in Tissues Other Than Brain in Alzheimer's Disease." *Nature* 341, no. 6239 (1989): 226–30.

King, Dana E., et al. "The Status of Baby Boomers' Health in the United States: The Healthiest Generation?" *JAMA Internal Medicine* 173, no. 5 (2013): 385–86.

King, Jaime, and Benjamin Moulton. " Group Health's Participation in a Shared Decision-Making Demonstration Yielded Lessons, Such as Role of Culture Change." *Health Affairs* 32, no. 2 (2013): 294–302.

Koepsell, Thomas D., et al. "Footwear Style and Risk of Falls in Older Adults." *Journal of the American Geriatrics Society* 52, no. 9 (2004): 1495–1501.

Kubler-Ross, Elisabeth. *On Death and Dying.* New York: Macmillan, 1969.

Lacey, Heather P., Dylan M. Smith, and Peter A. Ubel. "Hope I Die before I Get Old: Mispredicting Happiness across the Adult Lifespan," *Journal of Happiness Studies* 7 (2006): 167–82.

Larson, Eric B., and Robert A. Bruce. "Exercise and Aging." *Annals of Internal Medicine* 105 (1986): 783–85.

Larson Eric B., et al. "Adverse Drug Reactions Associated with Global Cognitive Impairment in Elderly Persons." *Annals of Internal Medicine* 107 (1987): 169–73.

———. "Exercise Is Associated with Reduced Risk for Incident Dementia among Persons 65 Years of Age and Older." *Annals of Internal Medicine* 144 (2006): 73–81.

Lautenschlager, Nicola, et al. "Effect of Physical Activity on Cognitive Function in Older Adults at Risk for Alzheimer Disease: A Randomized Trial." *JAMA* 300, no. 9 (2008): 1027–37.

Li, Fuzhong, et al. "Tai Chi and Fall Reductions in Older Adults: A Randomized Controlled Trial." *Journal of Gerontology: Medical Sciences* 60, no. 2 (2005): 187–94.

Lim, Alfredo, et al. "Clinico-neuropathological Correlation of Alzheimer's Disease in a Community-Based Case Series." *Journal of the American Geriatrics Society* 47, no. 5 (1999): 564–69.

Mafi, John N. et al. "Worsening Trends in the Management and Treatment of Back Pain." *JAMA Internal Medicine* 173, no. 17 (2013): 1573–81.

Martin, Douglas. "Robert A. Bruce Is Dead at 87; Pioneer of Cardiac Stress Test." *New York Times*, February 14, 2004.

McCullough, Dennis. *My Mother, Your Mother: Embracing "Slow Medicine," the Compassionate Approach to Caring for Your Aging Loved Ones.* New York City: HarperCollins, 2008.

———. "Slow Medicine." *Dartmouth Medicine*, Spring 2008.

Meier, Emily A., et al. "Defining a Good Death (Successful Dying): Literature Review and a Call for Research and Public Dialogue." *American Journal of Geriatric Psychiatry* 24, no 4 (2016): 261–71.

Moceri, Victoria, et al. "Using Census Data and Birth Certificates to Reconstruct the Early-Life Socioeconomic Environment and the Relation to the Development of Alzheimer's Disease." *Epidemiology* 12 (2001): 383–89.

Morris, Joan K., Derek G. Cook, and A. Gerald Shaper. "Loss of Employment and Mortality." *BMJ* 308, no. 6937 (1994): 1135–39.

Moynihan, Ray, and Alan Cassels. *Selling Sickness: How the World's Biggest Pharmaceutical Companies Are Turning Us All into Patients.* New York City: Nation Books, 2005.

Mozaffarian, Dariush, et al. "Executive Summary: Heart Disease and Stroke Statistics—2016 Update: A Report from the American Heart Association." *Circulation* 133 (2016): 447–54.

National Center for Complementary and Integrative Health. "Use of Complementary Health Approaches in the United States: National Health Interview Survey." https://nccih.nih.gov/research/statistics/NHIS/2012/mind-body/yoga.

National Center for Health Statistics. *Health, United States, 2015: With Special Feature on Racial and Ethnic Health Disparities.* Hyattsville, MD: National Center for Health Statistics, 2016.

National Heart, Lung, and Blood Institute. "Description of the DASH Eating Plan." https://www.nhlbi.nih.gov/health/health-topics/topics/dash.

National Institute on Deafness and Other Communication Disorders. "Age-Related Hearing Loss." https://www.nidcd.nih.gov/sites/default/files/Documents/health/hearing/AgeRelatedHearingLoss_0.pdf.

National Public Radio. "Is Preventive Medicine Actually Overtreatment?" *Science Friday*, February 11, 2011. http://www.npr.org/2011/02/11/133686016/Is-Preventive-Medicine-Actually-Overtreatment.

Netburn, Deborah. "What Does It Mean to Have a 'Good Death'?" *Los Angeles Times*, April 1, 2016.

Niazi, Asfandyar Khan, and Shaharyar Khan Niazi. "Mindfulness-Based Stress Reduction: A Non-pharmacological Approach for Chronic Illnesses." *North American Journal of Medical Sciences* 3, no. 1 (2011): 20–23.

NIH Senior Health. "Long-Term Care." http://nihseniorhealth.gov/longtermcare/faq/faq6.html.

Nikolova, Milena, and Carol Graham. "Employment, Late-Life Work, Retirement, and Well-Being in Europe and the United States." *IZA Journal of European Labor Studies* 3, no. 5 (2014): 1–30.

O'Connor, Anahad. "Exercise and Setting Ease Alzheimer's Effects." *New York Times*, November 4, 2003.

O'Connor, Annette M., et al. "Decision Aids for People Facing Health Treatment or Screening Decisions." *Cochrane Database of Systematic Reviews*, no. 1 (2003).

Oeffinger, Kevin C., et al. "Breast Cancer Screening for Women at Average Risk: 2015 Guideline Update from the American Cancer Society." *JAMA* 314, no. 15 (2015): 1599–1614.

Ortman, Jennifer M., Victoria A. Velkoff, and Howard Hogan. "An Aging Nation: The Older Population in the United States." U.S. Census Bureau, Current Population Reports P25-1140, May 2014, 1.

Our Bodies, Ourselves. "History." http://www.ourbodiesourselves.org/history/.

Parker-Pope, Tara. "Overtreatment Is Taking a Harmful Toll." *New York Times*, August 27, 2012. http://well.blogs.nytimes.com/2012/08/27/overtreatment-is-taking-a-harmful-toll/?_r=0.

Parson, Melissa, and Rebecca Hughes. "Three (Amazing) Group Health Patients Tell Stories of Participating in Our Research." Group Health Research Institute, April 22, 2016. https://www.grouphealthresearch.org/news-and-events/blog/2016/april/watch-our-new-video-group-health-research-made-real/.

PerryUndem Research/Communication. "Physicians' Views toward Advance Care Planning and End-of-Life Care Conversations: Findings from a National Survey among Physicians Who Regularly Treat Patients 65 and Older." Cambia Health Foundation, April 2016.

Pizzo, Philip A., and David M. Walker. "Should We Practice What We Profess? Care Near the End of Life." *New England Journal of Medicine* 372, no. 7 (2015): 595–98.

Rohwedder, Susann, and Robert J. Willis. "Mental Retirement." *Journal of Economic Perspectives: A Journal of the American Economic Association* 24, no. 1 (2010): 119–38.

Rosenberg, Dori E., et al. "The Feasibility of Reducing Sitting Time in Overweight and Obese Older Adults." *Health Education and Behavior* 42, no. 5 (2015): 669–76.

Roses Allen. "On the Discovery of the Genetic Association of Apolipoprotein E Genotypes and Common Late-Onset Alzheimer Disease." *Journal of Alzheimer's Disease.* 9, no. 3 (2006): S361–66.

Rowe, John W., and Robert L. Kahn. "Successful Aging." *Gerontologist* 37 (1997): 433–40.

Saddique, Haroon. "One Hour of Activity Needed to Offset Harmful Effects of Sitting at a Desk." *Guardian*, July 27, 2016.

Schwandt, Hannes. "Unmet Aspirations as an Explanation for the Age U-Shape in Wellbeing." *Journal of Economic Behavior and Organization* 122 (2016): 75–87.

———. "Why So Many of Us Experience a Mid-Life Crisis." *Harvard Business Review*, April 20, 2015.

Sherman, Karen J., et al. "Comparing Yoga, Exercise, and a Self-Care Book for Chronic Low Back Pain: A Randomized, Controlled Trial." *Annals of Internal Medicine* 143 (2005): 849–56.

Silveira, Maria J., Wyndy Wiitala, and John Piette. "Advance Directive Completion by Elderly Americans: A Decade of Change." *Journal of the American Geriatrics Society* 62, no. 4 (2014): 706–10.

Skoog, Ingmar, et al. "A Population-Based Study of Dementia in 85-Year-Olds." *New England Journal of Medicine* 328, no. 3 (1993): 153–58.

Sonnen, Joshua, et al. "Neuropathology in the Adult Changes in Thought Study: A Review." *Journal of Alzheimer's Disease* 18 (2009): 703–11.

SPRINT Research Group. "A Randomized Trial of Intensive versus Standard Blood-Pressure Control." *New England Journal of Medicine* 373 (2015): 2103–16.

Stack, Steven J. "A Call to Action: Physicians Must Turn the Tide of the Opioid Epidemic." *AMA Wire*, February 17, 2016. http://www.ama-assn.org/ama/ama-wire/post/call-action-physicians-must-turn-tide-of-opioid-epidemic.

Staudinger, Ursula M., et al. "A Global View on the Effects of Work on Health in Later Life." *Gerontologist* 56, no. S2 (2016): 281–92.

Temel, Jennifer S., et al. "Early Palliative Care for Patients with Metastatic Non-small-cell Lung Cancer." *New England Journal of Medicine* 363, no. 8 (2010): 733–42.

Teno, Joan M., et al. "Change in End-of-Life Care for Medicare Beneficiaries: Site of Death, Place of Care, and Health Care Transitions in 2000, 2005, and 2009." *JAMA* 309, no. 5 (2013): 470–77.

Teri, Linda, Rebecca G. Logsdon, and Susan M. McCurry. "Exercise Interventions for Dementia and Cognitive Impairment: The Seattle Protocols." *Journal of Nutrition, Health & Aging* 12, no. 6 (2008): 391–94.

Teri, Linda, et al. "Exercise Plus Behavioral Management in Patients with Alzheimer Disease: A Randomized Controlled Trial." *JAMA* 290, no. 15 (2003): 2015–22.

Tobacco Control Research Branch of the National Cancer Institute. "The Rewards of Quitting." SmokeFree.gov. https://smokefree.gov/rewards-of-quitting.

U.S. Department of Health and Human Services. *The Health Consequences of Smoking—50 Years of Progress: A Report of the Surgeon General.* Atlanta: U.S. Department of Health and Human Services, Centers for Disease Control and Prevention, National Center for Chronic Disease Prevention and Health Promotion, Office on Smoking and Health, 2014.

U.S. Preventive Services Task Force. "Final Update Summary: Breast Cancer: Screening." http://www.uspreventiveservicestaskforce.org/Page/Document/UpdateSummaryFinal/ breast-cancer-screening1.

Verghese, Joe, et al. "Leisure Activities and the Risk of Dementia in the Elderly." *New England Journal of Medicine* 348, no. 25 (2003): 2508–16.

Von Korff, Michael, and Gary Franklin. "Responding to America's Iatrogenic Epidemic of Prescription Opioid Addiction and Overdose." *Medical Care* 54, no. 5 (2016): 426–29.

Voukelatos, Alexander, et al. "A Randomized, Controlled Trial of Tai Chi for the Prevention of Falls: The Central Sydney Tai Chi Trial." *Journal of the American Geriatrics Society* 55 (2007): 1185–91.

Wagner, Anita K., et al. "Benzodiazepine Use and Hip Fractures in the Elderly: Who Is at Greatest Risk?" *Archives of Internal Medicine* 164, no. 14 (2004): 1567–72.

Welch, H. Gilbert. "When Screening Is Bad for a Woman's Health." *Los Angeles Times*, July 19, 2015.

Welch, H. Gilbert, et al. "Breast-Cancer Tumor Size, Overdiagnosis, and Mammography Screening Effectiveness." *New England Journal of Medicine* 375, no. 15 (2016): 1438–47.

Willis, Sherry L., et al. "Long-Term Effects of Cognitive Training on Everyday Functional Outcomes in Older Adults." *JAMA* 296, no. 23 (2006): 2805–14.

Wolf, Steven L., et al. "Reducing Frailty and Falls in Older Persons: An Investigation of Tai Chi and Computerized Balance Training." *Journal of the American Geriatrics Society* 44, no. 5 (1996): 489–97.

Writing Group for the Women's Health Initiative Investigators. "Risks and Benefits of Estrogen Plus Progestin in Healthy Postmenopausal Women: Principal Results from the Women's Health Initiative Randomized Controlled Trial." *JAMA* 288, no. 3 (2002): 321–33.

Zubenko, George S., et al. "Family Study of Platelet Membrane Fluidity in Alzheimer's Disease." *Science* 238 (1987): 539–42.

INDEX

ABOUT THE AUTHORS

Eric B. Larson, MD, is a leading expert in the science of healthy aging. Since 1986, he has led a large, longitudinal research program focused on delaying and preventing Alzheimer's disease, other forms of dementia, and declines in memory and thinking. Called the Adult Changes in Thought (ACT) study, this program is the world's longest-running study of its kind and includes one of the largest research populations age 85 and older. Larson is also vice president for research and health care innovation for the Washington region of Kaiser Permanente (formerly Group Health) and executive director of Kaiser Permanente Washington Health Research Institute. In addition, he is a clinical professor of medicine at the University of Washington (UW) School of Medicine and of health services at the UW School of Public Health. He also maintains an internal-medicine practice, providing primary care to his patients since 1975. Before joining Group Health in 2002, Larson served as medical director for the UW Medical Center and associate dean for clinical affairs at its medical school from 1989 to 2002. He is a member and past president of the Society of General Internal Medicine; member and former chair of the Board of Regents of the American College of Physicians; a master of the American College of Physicians; and an elected member of the National Academy of Medicine (formerly called the Institute of Medicine) of the National Academy of Sciences. Larson has published hundreds of research papers in peer-review medical journals—including the *Journal of the American Medical Association*, the *New England Journal of Medicine*, and *Annals of Internal Medicine*.

Joan DeClaire is a journalist specializing in health, psychology, and family relationships. She is coauthor of three books with John Gottman, PhD: *Raising an Emotionally Intelligent Child: The Heart of Parenting* (1998); *The Relationship Cure: A 5-Step Guide to Strengthening Your Marriage, Family, and Friendships* (2002); and *Ten Lessons to Transform Your Marriage: America's Love Lab Experts Share Their Strategies for Strengthening Your Relationship* (2007). She currently works as director of communications at Kaiser Permanente Washington Health Research Institute.